Throw Me a Smile

Throw Me a Smile

Colleen Morgan

For my daughter and all of her angels
(and their mothers …)

Published by Moodie Media, 9 Brunswick Road, Ealing,
London W5 1BB, UK

ISBN 978-0-473-29645-2
Ebook ISBN 978-0-473-29844-9

To contact Colleen Morgan, email: ctmorgan@hol.gr
A percentage of proceeds from the sale of *Throw Me a Smile* will be
donated to Elpida, the Association of Friends of Children with Cancer
(www.elpida.org)

Editorial services by Oratia Media, www.oratiamedia.com

First published 2014
Printed in China by Nordica

Preface

21 January 2009

It has the makings of a normal mid-winter morning on Rhodes. The sky is clear Aegean blue, a magnificent colour that provides the perfect backdrop for the unique town in which I live. The breeze is fresh enough to have me upping the pace of my daily beachfront walk. The sea is rougher than normal, wild and uninviting, and the usual steady stream of winter swimmers have left the town's main beach disappointed this morning.

I find myself striding faster than usual, anxious to finish my daily circuit along the boulevard to the colourful Mandrake marina and town centre. To do what, I wonder? I haven't made any plans for the day so where is that anxious feeling coming from?

My hands are cold. I thrust them into my windbreaker pockets and feel my mobile buzzing.

I pull the phone out, at the same time reaching for my car keys without checking the caller ID. It's a woman. 'Oh, hello, good morning, is that Mrs Morgan? It's the assistant principal from the high school. I have your daughter in my office and she is not feeling well. She says she has a headache, her ears are aching and she really doesn't look well.

'Should I send her home or will you come and pick her up?

'Mrs Morgan, are you there? Can you hear me? I have your daughter here and she isn't feeling well ...'

Despite the slow morning traffic in downtown Rhodes I am outside Lucy's high school within minutes, banging my way through the heavy wrought-iron entrance gates and up the stairs to find my daughter.

She is with the assistant principal, who is a short, petite woman, with a face that shows her emotions. I've seen her tight-lipped and angry, tired of dealing with difficult teenagers, but this morning she is clearly troubled.

She sees I am shaken and says nothing as she puts her arm around Lucy's hunched shoulders, guiding her into my arms. We are out the door.

'What's wrong?'

'It's my head, my nose, my ears.' Lucy shrugs. She is still quiet an hour later as we check into the island's new medical centre for an emergency scan that has been hastily arranged by her doctor.

The young technician is reassuring. 'It will only take 30 minutes or so. Go and take a seat outside and your daughter will be out in no time.'

I find a space in the cramped, cheerless waiting room. I try to chat to the other patients and quickly realise that their appointments have been arranged weeks in advance. Lucy's scan is disrupting their schedule.

They have already been waiting a long time in that confined antechamber and, as the minutes slowly tick by, their impatience surfaces.

'What's taking so long?'

'What's your daughter having done in there? How can you sit there for so long and not ask questions?'

I look at them and feel as if someone else is shaking my head. I check the clock; an hour and 20 minutes have passed and a feeling of dread floods my stomach.

'She'll be out soon,' I tell them. 'They know what they are looking for and Lucy knows as well …'

1

The summer of 2001 was much like any other summer on Rhodes. It was hot and the island was busy, packed with holidaymakers, all enjoying the sunshine, the beaches and the sights that make Rhodes one of the most sought-after destinations in the Mediterranean.

I was in the upmarket Old Town Gallery where I'd worked for the past five summer seasons. My job? Sales, talking wealthy Americans into buying pieces of jewellery they probably didn't really want and certainly didn't need.

My customers were always surprised to find a New Zealander working in a shop in the walled medieval town, many quick to pry into my past with questions about my background, my family and why I had settled on the island. To be honest, I rarely wanted to give away too many details, especially then. It had been a difficult year; a separation from the man who had changed my life, a rushed trip back to New Zealand because my mother was ill and the usual money problems. It wasn't over yet.

I don't think my four children noticed. They were still enjoying their summer holidays. Yanni, 16 and the oldest of the foursome, should have been working. Instead he spent most of the long summer days on the beach, flirting with the pretty local girls and training for the kayak nationals. My 14-year-old twins, Tony and Sam, no longer children but not yet young men, were bursting with enthusiasm, ideas, laughter and cheek. They kept busy with their mates, on the beach, playing volleyball, skateboarding; doing boys' things.

Their bouncy, blonde tomboy sister, Lucy, also spent a lot of time on the beach, swimming, playing, and enjoying her friends' company.

Her name is really Lucia May. She was named after her two grandmothers: Lucia, my Greek-Italian mother-in-law who was a daily part of Lucy's upbringing, and my mother, May, the soft-spoken Nana who lives on the other side of the world, in my home town of Christchurch.

After three boys, I hadn't considered having another child. In fact I'd had a coil fitted. However, Lucy arrived, the full stop to the family, a strong-willed, sturdy little character who ran like the wind and already, at seven, swam like a dolphin. She was a handful, fighting and cursing alongside her brothers. She treasured her dolls and was well behaved at school.

Lucy liked to be at the centre of things without always being the centre of attention. She loved games and mischief, and she also liked her food. Every time she passed the gallery on her way to the beach she was eating: crisps, chocolates, anything unhealthy, by the bag full. My comments to watch what she was eating, to look after her teeth, brought nothing more than a cheeky grin and a shake of her blonde curls as she ran out the side door towards her friends. Lucy was what Mum called a bonnie baby, a rounded and well-built child, never thin, always fit and healthy looking.

During that summer she put on a few kilos. The twins teased and scoffed at her cellulite and Lucy reddened, pulling at her swimming costume, which suddenly was one size too small. I noticed that her appetite was changing, though; she was picky and showed little interest in food. I thought she was tired of the boys' taunts about her chubby image and didn't pay too much attention to her habits. She was moodier as well, seemed to yell a lot and started to complain of earache.

I booked an appointment with a local ear, nose and throat specialist. When the time came to leave the house Lucy was nowhere to be seen; she was off in the Old Town of Rhodes with her mischievous young friends. Anxious, I wandered the cobbled streets and alleys, calling into pebbled courtyards, knocking on the heavy doors of the old homes, until she turned up full of high spirits and the fast food souvlaki they had just eaten.

The earache had gone, cured by laughter and good company.

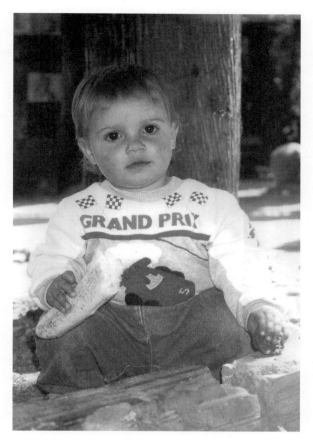

A bonnie child: Lucy in her element
with bread, biscuit and bricks

It returned a week or so later, along with a blocked nose that produced heavy mucus that never seemed to clear, and a swelling on the side of her neck. I took her to an ear, nose and throat specialist, whose surgery resembled a recording studio, with unusual music and recording certificates outnumbering the more mundane medical diplomas on the walls. This ENT expert was quick, examining Lucy's neck, her throat and her ears.

'Everything is fine,' he said, 'and don't worry about the lump. It will disappear in a couple of months.'

He wrote a prescription for antibiotics and called in the next patient.

Two weeks later, Lucy and I paid him another visit. The antibiotics were gone but the earache and the blocked nose remained. He tested her hearing, touched the lump and reassured me.

'It's nothing, don't worry.'

Somehow his words weren't as comforting the second time. His smile and easygoing manner clashed with Lucy's pale face and sad, troubled eyes. I suggested a blood test, just to ease my mind.

'Good idea,' he said and off we went. The results showed she had an infection.

'The ear, of course,' he said.

We were getting nowhere. More antibiotics. Lucy vomited at school. I needed a second opinion so we went to Lucy's paediatrician, who was more concerned with the lump on her neck than her ear infection. He recommended another blood test and more antibiotics.

Lucy lost interest in school, preferring the couch to her friends' company during the afternoon hours. At night she tossed in a restless sleep and her heavy snoring kept me awake. I was discouraged and concerned about the antibiotics and the lack of results.

One morning she struggled to wake and she somehow didn't look like Lucy. She was pale, strangely quiet and reserved. Until I said there would be no school and that we would be going to the doctors again. Then all hell was let loose. Lucy went wild and our cramped house was not big enough to contain her fury.

Screaming and crying, she knew that something was wrong. I wondered if it was fear or hatred that flashed in her eyes. She cursed me for dragging her into the doctor's surgery and loathed me even more when the specialist quietly suggested time in hospital.

'To clear the lump,' he explained to Lucy. 'It will only take a few days and then you will be back with your friends again. You'll see, Lucy.'

It took some time to return home from his surgery to pack a small bag for the hospital. My only sharp memory was of Lucy's face, a mind's snapshot of a little girl scared out of her wits.

After the inevitable paperwork, Lucy was admitted to the children's ward of the new Rhodes hospital, an impressive building on the outskirts of the town, with a fine view over the sea towards the coast of Turkey and the small island of Symi that Lucy and I had visited with friends earlier that summer. We had enjoyed 24 hours of laughter, giggles and

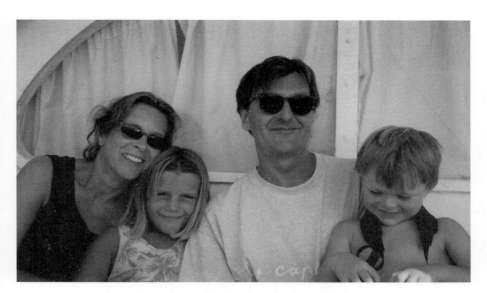

Returning to Rhodes from Symi with Chris,
John and Henry, midsummer 2001

surprises. My London friends, Chris and John, had booked us into a small hotel behind the harbour area. It was last minute; the island was busy as it was the height of the season. Our room was cramped and airless but Lucy and I pretended it was a luxury suite. We dined on lobster and shrimp. I enjoyed fine wine and cocktails while Lucy played with my friends' son, Henry, coaxing the younger boy into the crystal-clear water, teasing him into more daring swimming and diving. Lucy and Henry had been a delight together, sharing summer laughter and excitement.

As Lucy and I settled into the sterile hospital room with a view of a helicopter pad, that weekend seemed a lifetime ago. First impressions, however, weren't so bad; Lucy had company with other children and, as always, made friends quickly and easily. With friends and relatives there during visiting hours the room was rarely empty and, initially, the hours and days passed comfortably enough.

The nursing staff and doctors, many of whom I knew from previous hospital visits with the boys, quickly began a series of tests and examinations; I was confident that they would find what was troubling Lucy. A good vein was found in her right hand, which was bandaged into a bulky, protective, bat-shaped mitten, her tiny palm supported by a piece of wood to prevent any damage to the intravenous butterfly clip that ensured painless blood tests. More antibiotics were prescribed and a dreadful waiting game began.

On the third day Lucy packed her clothes, books and bags. She'd had enough and, after all, as she was quick to point out, her doctor had said three days was all it would take.

We didn't leave, however, and the tests and the medicines and the waiting continued.

A week and many blood, urine, allergy tests and ultrasonic scans later, the doctors remained puzzled. They were noncommittal when I asked what the tests showed. 'Be patient. We know what we are doing so don't concern yourself with things that you don't understand,' they said.

I told them it wasn't just the swelling. Lucy also continued to suffer from a blocked nose; she had stopped eating; she was distraught and anxious, and distrustful of any nurses and staff in white coats. The vein in her right hand was damaged; her left hand had been bandaged for tests until that too proved useless.

'I'm sick of having needles stuck into me,' Lucy told them. 'I don't want to be prodded and poked any more.

'I want to go home.'

Wednesday 5 December 2001

Lucy didn't go home. She remained in Rhodes Hospital, a wary withdrawn little patient, with me constantly at her bedside. Not that I wanted to be elsewhere, but mothers or carers did not choose to stay with their patients, it was expected. The days were long and the evenings and nights endless as I fought to sleep on the adjacent bed or on the uncomfortable chair next to Lucy's bed.

I didn't sleep at all last night after the arrival of a two-month old baby whose young mother refused to turn off the light. It was the first time Lucy herself asked me to sleep with her.

This morning my stomach was tight, knotted.

I called my sister-in-law, a midwife who lived in Athens, to check out a cat scratch allergy test that the hospital had supposedly sent away to the mainland days ago.

The director of the children's ward had told me the results would be available in ten days. I asked him again.

'It's no big thing. We'll wait a week or so for those results and then see what we can do,' he said to his audience of young female nurses. Pulling at the immaculate camel hair coat on his shoulders, he turned sharply on expensive brogues, and high headed his way out of the ward as if he was leading a fashion parade and not the morning rounds of frightened young patients.

In her usual rather sharp telephone style, my sister-in-law, Maria, told me to get out of the hospital, no matter what.

'Leave now,' she said, 'and bring Lucy immediately to Athens.'

I swallowed hard hearing her tone; it was an order rather than a request, but Maria wasn't abrupt, she sounded scared. I went to the director, who insisted I ignore Maria's suggestion.

'Your child should stay here,' he said, his defiant stare daring me to overrule. I felt tired, drained, close to tears and stripped of confidence. Maria's words pounded through my brain. 'Get her out of there.'

I hadn't noticed the arrival of the hospital social worker, but she appeared, a guardian angel, just when I was starting to lose it and a defiant Lucy, frightened and confused, definitely was not willing to listen to me.

She did listen to Mary, who was an extraordinary lady with a very special manner and an aura that calmed us both down. Mary had a Madonna smile, soothing, strong and mesmerising. I felt her warm, deep brown eyes looking in to my muddled thoughts, reading my insecurity and fear. In her face I found the assurance and strength I was lacking.

Mary spoke to Lucy about the need to put a name to whatever it was that was making her ill in order to cure it, and of the possibility of a trip to Athens to meet with specialists. She spoke to me of my uncertainty and my unwillingness to go against the hospital system and she advised me to follow my instincts.

'Do what's best for your daughter. You're a mother, a good, caring mother, you know what you must do and, don't worry, you will find the strength to do whatever is needed.'

She left the ward and so did we.

No more second thoughts. I packed our things and we walked out of the hospital without the director's blessing, without any official referral papers, without the test results. The only support, apart from sympathetic glances from the nursing staff and withdrawn younger doctors probably wary of the director's wrath, came from the assistant director.

Dina had been part of the spectacle of the twins' birth 14 years previously, when I found myself whisked away for an emergency caesarean with 12 doctors and their trainees vying for the best view in the operating theatre. She always remembered the boys and always asked after 'our' twins. She was a strong, no-nonsense lady, someone you could rely on. She handed me an envelope. 'Give this to the doctors in Athens. It's not much but at least they will have some idea of the tests we have done here.'

We went home to shower and to make hurried preparations for the trip to Athens. I called Lucy's father and told him I was taking his sister's advice and going to Athens. He was quiet and non-committal. Since our separation almost a year ago we had spoken rarely; I didn't want Yorgos back in my life but our problems had to be shelved. I booked flights to Athens and arranged for my mother-in-law to stay with the boys in the Old Town until our return.

At midday the boys bounded in from school, happy and excited to see Lucy and me home, their enthusiasm dashed, slapped from their faces when they heard we were booked to fly to Athens later in the evening.

They were followed by Lucy's school friends, clambering at the back door, their noisy enthusiasm and smiles turning to grave little frowns as they realised their friend was not home to stay.

I wanted to clean, check the damp corners of the hall, ensure the cupboards were full, and sort the bills. I was all over the place, lost, muddled and alone.

I hadn't time to concentrate on Lucy's feelings and the moment I did I found myself blinking heavily, blinking back tears to clear the image of a frightened little girl who was my daughter.

Lucy had a few moments to enjoy her brothers and her friends. In the evening we boarded a flight to Athens. At first Lucy was anxious and irritable, showing no confidence in herself, and little more in me. She did, however, enjoy the flight, a new experience, and an hour-long interlude of pampering by the young flight attendants; in the air Lucy forgot her problems and laughed. My beautiful little blonde with the infectious giggle and sparkling eyes was back, but not for long.

Maria and her husband, George, met us at the huge new Eleftherios Venizelos Athens Airport, a bustling crossroad from Europe into the Middle East, Asia and beyond. Lucy was quiet and conversation was limited as we drove to their new home, their escape from the bustle and pollution of downtown Athens.

Maria and George started their married life together in the early

1980s in an apartment within walking distance of central Athens and its magnificent Acropolis. That source of dreams for holidaymakers and historians could be a nightmare for its residents who faced increasing problems of congestion, overcrowding, noise and pollution. Looking for a better quality of life, Maria and George, who was a major in the Greek army, invested out of the city, their new home looking towards the lights of the throbbing capital in the distance.

As George fussed over his niece, the only girl in the 'family' of three brothers and three male cousins, and Maria prepared an evening meal, I thought how their large house, the top of three levels built into the Anthousa hillside, contrasted to my pokey little home. Their house spoke of their success; did mine speak of my failure?

Maria explained that she had spoken to a surgeon at the Agia (Saint) Sofia Paidon (Children's) Hospital and had arranged a meeting with him in the morning. Any other conversation was slow and laboured, curbed by our weariness and thoughts of what lay ahead.

Lucy and I slept together in her cousin's bed.

Thursday 6 December

Up very early and Lucy was not interested in getting out of bed; I couldn't blame her, as neither of us knew what was in store.

George drove us into a freezing cold, austere Athens to wait for more than an hour in a pokey locker room at the women's hospital Maria worked in. Her colleagues were warm and friendly, welcoming Lucy with hot chocolate and pastries that remained untouched. We took a taxi to the Saint Sofia Children's Hospital for a meeting with Dr Dolatza who, if necessary, would operate on Lucy's neck.

A quietly spoken, middle-aged man with a caring face, the surgeon checked Lucy's neck and chatted to her, and before either of us realised what was happening, we were led from his office to a busy outpatients waiting area into a sea of mothers and children of all ages, one crying, one coughing, another demanding attention. Bedlam!

Fortunately Lucy was promptly seen by another doctor, who checked her throat and neck and told us she would have to stay in the hospital for tests. The paperwork was straightforward, Lucy was officially admitted into that busy bustling hospital, and we were directed to the lift to the sixth floor. The lift, with its old concertina door and noisy creaking chamber, was like the hospital in general – a shock after Rhodes. It all seemed so old and grey and worn down.

On the sixth floor we were shown to a crowded room with at least eight beds in it. I took a deep breath and felt Lucy's hand squeezing, pulling down on mine. There were beds and chairs, children, mothers and grandmothers everywhere. It was cramped, stifling and claustrophobic.

Maria told us to wait and hurried off down the corridor. Neither Lucy nor I wanted to sit in that room. We found a stark lounge area where a young intern was working. For a while it was just the three of us in that grey, colourless room of tables and chairs, the doctor oblivious to our intrusion.

More people came into the lounge. Lucy chatted to a young couple that had, she discovered, honeymooned on Rhodes. They were awaiting test results on their three-month-old daughter. The mum commented on Lucy's good manners, her intelligence and her easy rapport with adults. She assured her she would be returning home soon.

Another young girl, all smiles and freckles, her light brown hair pulled back into two untidy pigtails, bounded into the room, her bright pyjamas a rainbow against the grey walls. 'Hi, I'm Yorgia, I'm 12, well, nearly 13 really,' she said to Lucy. 'One of the nurses just told me that you might have had a reaction from a cat scratch.'

Yorgia told Lucy about a lump she had in her armpit. 'No big deal,' she said, her grin all confidence. 'I had an operation and the lump's gone now and I'm going home tomorrow. You'll see, they will do a whole lot of tests and yours will be the same. Don't be sad,' she added, smiling at Lucy's worried face, 'this place isn't so bad, and I've made a lot of new friends here. I have to go now, bye!' Yorgia hurried off down the corridor.

I wondered who had told her about Lucy's lump. Seemed news travelled fast on the ward.

Lunch was offered but Lucy was not tempted by anything on the brown plastic tray. Not that I blamed her. At least my comment that all the Greek hospitals must rely on the same cook brought a smile.

'That's why the food was always cold in Rhodes,' she chuckled. 'It had to make a long journey before it reached us.'

Lucy's smile disappeared with the soft footsteps of an approaching nurse. The nurse led us along the corridor to another much smaller room, with three beds. She pointed to an empty bed by the window and closed the door.

It seemed that we had been upgraded. Maria must have been shocked at the state of the larger room as well; I presumed she was using her hospital contacts to ensure that her niece was in comfortable surroundings.

We were introduced to a pretty young woman, Elpida, and her daughter, Eleni, from Mytilini, and another girl with a small, three-and-a-half-year-old son who seemed much, much younger. Lucy settled on her bed and within minutes was called for a CT scan and an x-ray. On the way down to the ground floor the slender blonde doctor who had spoken to me earlier, asking for the details of Lucy's family and short medical history, explained that Lucy would be having an exploratory operation the following day to find the cause of the swelling. 'I haven't been given many details, but the surgeon will cut into the side of your daughter's neck to examine what's causing the problem. He'll probably use the surgery to take something for a biopsy.'

She checked my startled face, adding quickly, 'But that's standard procedure, nothing out of the ordinary. I believe your sister-in-law is talking with the surgeon again so she may be able to tell you more.'

She guided us through a heavy door and left us to wait for Lucy to be called for the scan. Thank God Maria was doing most of the talking; she worked daily with doctors, she knew the hospital system and was using her contacts to move Lucy through quickly.

The scan was reasonably straightforward, although a bit of a shock at first for both of us. Lucy was shown into a room dominated by a large box-like machine with a hole, a short tunnel, in the middle. It looked a bit like the front of a flat camera. She was told to lie down on a narrow examination table while a nurse injected fluid into her arm. At first she nodded assent and said nothing but her eyes told me she was scared.

'Okay Loukia. We are ready to start now,' the nurse explained. 'Mrs Mortzou, please wait outside. The test won't take very long.'

Lucy started to sob. 'Mum, don't leave me in here!'

The nurse turned quickly to Lucy and asked her to remain calm. 'It's all right. Your mother can stay with you but she will have to put that on,' she said, pointing to a heavy protective apron. So I stayed, weighed down by that hefty garment, as the machine moved and clicked over Lucy's head, neck and chest.

She did exactly as she was told, remaining dead still as time seemed to pass only with the slow rhythm of the scanner. I had time to think. I was protected from the radiation in that room but wondered what protection Lucy had. I felt useless, realising I was totally ignorant of this type of procedure, which was nothing like the ultrasounds I'd had during pregnancy. I resolved to learn about them online as soon as we returned to Rhodes, but that didn't help my feeling of ineptitude.

Back on the ward I couldn't sleep, couldn't relax. The room was small and cramped and Lucy was very much against sharing her bed. I sat upright in the uncomfortable chair until she fell asleep and then I lay on her bed anyway, curling along the bottom, her toes for company.

I had no other choice.

Friday 7 December

Lucy was not allowed any food or fluids from midnight in preparation for the operation to relieve the swelling on her neck and possibly take tissue for a biopsy. She was scared of the doctors, hated being jabbed and was constantly telling them and the nurses about her treatment in the hospital in Rhodes.

'They jabbed and pricked at me all the time,' she explained to each nurse who came into the room. 'Look what they did to my hand, they didn't care for me,' she said, sobbing back the big tears that streamed down her cheeks.

Maria's arrival this morning coincided with the appearance of a young nurse. 'Hi Lucia. I have to take you to see another doctor, an ear, nose and throat specialist. That's a mouthful isn't it?' she said, smiling into Lucy's eyes. Lucy reluctantly took her outstretched hand, reaching back to entwine her tiny fingers in mine as the nurse led us out of the room and down a long corridor. Swing doors were pushed open, left to flap noisily behind us as we passed by anonymous offices and numbered doors until one opened and a white-coated doctor ushered us quickly inside.

A tall man, hair greying at the temples, leaned over me and told me to sit with Lucy, to hold her in a chair.

'But she can sit by herself!'

'No, you must hold her, like this,' he said, pushing us down on to the chair and crossing my arms across Lucy's waist.

'Tight. Hold her tight.'

He bent down and, without any explanation or warning, fed a small tube with a light on the end up her nose. It was done so quickly that we were both shocked into complying. Lucy panicked and started to scream as blood splattered her nightgown.

I was shocked. It was as if my little girl had been violated. I was speechless and Maria was a deathly white. The doctor removed his glasses, tapping the frame against his front teeth in a moment of thought. 'One of her tonsils isn't moving … there's a spot at the back of her throat.'

There was an atmosphere of trouble, doom.

As Lucy left the chair, shaken and shocked, her new pink nightgown, a hasty gift from her closest friend in Rhodes, splattered with blood, she faced the doctor, bit her lip, dropped her head and apologised. 'Sorry. I'm sorry I screamed. I'm sorry that I made such a fuss.'

Stifling a sob, she lifted her head to look at the doctor and she thanked him. I felt like hitting the man. I opened my mouth to speak but there was no opportunity to ask any questions. As quickly as we had been ushered into the room, we were shown out and the door closed behind us.

We returned to our room, 676, and I quickly tried to change Lucy's soiled nightdress. A nurse offered us a green surgical gown.

Panic hit my stomach and I did my best to fight it back. Lucy looked threatened, angered and lost. Even smaller, she seemed to be shrinking by the minute, so precious, so frail.

A male nurse or orderly banged open the door, wheeling in a trolley bed, ready, he said, to take Lucy to surgery. Lucy screamed and he left.

We had a couple of minutes to calm down before Lucy, her aunt and I walked hand-in-hand to the lift and went down to the first floor. I felt awful, dry-mouthed and useless.

As a threesome we moved through the heavy swing doors marked 'Surgery'. To the right a woman called Lucy's name and spoke softly to her. Only one of us was allowed to remain and Lucy opted for her aunt.

I wanted to object but found myself swept through the surgery doors by a nurse. The door shut behind me and Maria followed seconds later.

My friend Cecilia, who had been a colleague in Rhodes but now lived in Athens, was somehow by my side, squeezing my hand, asking what was going on. I tried to talk to my kind-hearted Philippine friend but no words formed. I could only shrug and give a strange sigh.

It was just before 1pm. We started to wait.

I was standing, leaning against the wall, holding Lucy's slippers. It was easy at first. Cecilia and I chatted, small talk and gossip about Rhodes and the people she and her family had left behind to settle in Athens. Cecilia was bright and reassuring. Her eyes told me she was hurting, hurting for me, and hurting for Lucy.

The minutes slipped by and tears glazed my eyes. I started to shake and tremble. I was cold and I was afraid of what they were going to do to my little girl.

Cecilia left and I realised that Lucy had been behind those doors for more than an hour. Other children seemed to reappear quickly, but not Lucy. 'Calm down, Coll,' I told myself. 'The doctor told you the operation would be exploratory, nothing to worry about … but I should have asked for more details.'

My eyes locked with Maria's. She was getting anxious as well.

I was unaware of the tears that lined my cheeks until the salty taste reached my lips. I thought of all the times that I'd been angry with Lucy. The times we'd argued, when I'd told her what a horrible child she was. I regretted every word. Biopsy. The word tore its way through my thoughts. 'Calm down. The doctor said the biopsy was mandatory.'

My niece, Tania, and my father were suddenly in my thoughts; it was almost as if they were next to me. Were they there to help me, to give me strength? Or were they preparing me for the worst? That really hadn't entered my head.

Tania, my beautiful niece, was my family's first grandchild. Part Maori on her father's side, she had gorgeous chocolate-brown skin, huge questioning eyes and a throw-back-your-head laugh. Tania's head, however, was too big; she had suffered convulsions and died of a massive brain tumour shortly after her fourth birthday, when I was 13. She had never walked, she uttered only a few words, and she had been wild and difficult at times but God, how she'd adored my father, who had danced with her, singing her favourite song until her eyes shone and his own eyes had filled with tears. Dad.

The kind, strong gentleman I was fortunate enough to call my father died when I was pregnant with the twins. Before retiring from the local hospital board in the late 1970s he had fought for a revolutionary change in standard hospital equipment, ensuring that patients with terminal cancer were given comfortable, bright rooms with nice furnishings and a television.

'You're the end of the rainbow, you're my pot of gold,
Daddy's little girl, to have and to hold …'

My hand in his, he had whispered fragments of my favourite childhood song the night before he passed away. Jack Morgan died in one of his comfortable rooms, succumbing to a cancer that had plagued him since his return to New Zealand from fighting in Egypt during the Second World War.

I blinked back to the present as the surgery doors banged open. The surgeon was positive; he mentioned lymph glands and tonsils. 'Lucy's fine, she's just coming out of the anaesthetic.' He patted my shoulder and said the ear, nose and throat specialist had caused the delay. 'Wait here for your daughter. She'll be out in a minute and will be looking for you.'

He turned to Maria and they started down the stairs towards his office. I stood by the heater, aware of its warmth, but I couldn't stop shaking. For the first time I was conscious of the other people waiting by the surgery doors.

Had they been there all along?

Some were chatting, their hands wrapped around throwaway polystyrene coffee cups; others looked how I felt, lost and bewildered, each deep in their own thoughts and fears.

Ten minutes dragged by and Maria returned. The initial biopsy, she said, was good, and I felt a warm wave of relief run through my body.

Then Lucy was out of the theatre, her bed pushed through the doors; she was awake and she was smiling. Her face banished my fears. I felt light-headed, elated, relieved.

Somehow we were back in 676 and Lucy was drowsy but fine. A doctor came to add a plaster to the side of Lucy's neck and she slept. She stirred, woke suddenly, her nose bloody, and vomited, a horrible bloody brown substance, then slept again.

Maria and George came by to check on their niece. They had spoken again with the surgeon and told me that some glands had been removed but Lucy's tonsils had not been touched; the biopsy reports, they assured me, were good.

Relief.

Thank you God. Thank you Saint Nicholas, whoever got her through that nasty surgery, thank you!

Saturday 8 December

Lucy woke early after a restless night. She wasn't in pain and went to the toilet, which pleased the nurses. Maria was in early, as was as Dr Dolatza. We talked briefly about the tooth that Lucy had taken out earlier in the summer.

'That could have had something to do with the swelling,' he said. He left me thinking about that troublesome tooth. It had grown up instead of down, and had wound its way into Lucy's gums like an octopus and ultimately had tested the expertise of the Athenian specialist who had been called in to take it out. He had told me that he had never seen anything like it.

Lucy had been more than two hours in the dentist's chair, and I had paced the floor, struggling to cope with my daughter's cries and pleas to go home. She had screamed in fear and pain as the effects of the initial injection wore off and they had injected again and again until they had won the battle. She looked shattered and was white with rage and fear.

Minutes later she walked into the surgery and thanked the dentist, just as she had the ear, nose and throat specialist. In both cases she had thanked and hugged the men that I could happily have hit.

A strange reaction from her, but both men had smiled.

I was jolted from my thoughts by the young doctor we had seen in the lounge area the previous day. Seemingly unaware of the other children in the room, he checked Lucy and gave her a kiss on the cheek.

She smiled and said that the doctors in Rhodes would never have done that.

Another doctor, a petite well-dressed woman, her white overcoat flapping to show meticulously matched work clothes, entered the room. It seemed that all the attention was on Lucy as no one acknowledged the other children. This doctor was preoccupied, her eyes straining to focus on Lucy's chart through tiny bifocals. She didn't even look up when she asked Lucy's height and weight.

I moved closer to ask what was happening, but her look was enough to make me shut my mouth. I felt like I had been slapped. An older doctor entered, or rather, barged in. I will never forget her sweeping past Elpida and Eleni in a huge green surgery gown that was tied at the waist like a bag. She and the smaller doctor whispered together before turning to me.

'Pack up your daughter's things. Come along Lucy, we are off to another room, much nicer than this, with a television and bright curtains.'

Strange, I thought, mentioning those things in that cold grey hospital.

Suddenly something hit, connecting my most chilling fears and thoughts. For a split second I was back in the Christchurch hospital room with Dad, moments before he passed away.

I didn't have time to dwell on it.

The big woman with the billowing surgery gown was talking to me, at me. She was impatient, unnerving. 'Come with us. We have to talk.'

I followed the doctors into their office and started to freeze, to shake uncontrollably. Shivering, I tried to speak. My Greek had gone and not even English words came out. The oversized woman in green was saying something about cancerous cells that had to be stopped. She was talking about my Lucy, my little girl who had just gone through horrible surgery, a pale little girl who used to be scared of nothing and now hated doctors and screamed at the sight of needles.

I was shaking so much I couldn't hear well. I must have been crying as the smaller doctor offered me a tissue. I tried to breathe properly, tried desperately to think and concentrate on what this woman was saying. I had to talk to Lucy's surgeon. He had told me just an hour or so earlier that it was all to do with her tooth.

I felt stifled, choked, and I couldn't focus. My mobile rattled in my hand as I tried to call Maria, until the doctor whisked it away to talk in the corridor, away from me.

'What's happening?'

'Go to your room and wait,' she said, adding something about Maria living too far away.

'This is all taking too long', she said impatiently. 'I should have been gone long ago.'

I wanted to hit her, tug out what little strange hair she had but I wasn't capable of doing anything. Save pray. Pray that this was just another muddled dream, like all the others I'd been having lately; pray that I would wake and thank God that it was simply a dream. We would be back in Rhodes, laughing at home, doing something stupid, anything, anywhere but in this hospital.

Never had I felt so alone, desperate and abandoned.

My in-laws arrived with Saki, their eldest son who was 19 and Lucy's godfather. Saki quickly filled the chair beside Lucy's bed, tucking his legs under her bed to get as close as possible to his godchild. He took control of the room, his bright chatter and easy smile breaking the cold, deadly atmosphere. Lucy was laughing at his antics as I headed to the door.

Lucy's surgeon reappeared. Had he been here all along? Why didn't he talk to me again? I felt Maria and George guiding me along the corridor.

What's wrong with me?

I was in a daze as we passed the nurses' station, concerned eyes following us along the corridor. Through heavy doors we moved into another wing on the same floor and turned left into a quieter clinic and sat on the edge of uncomfortable chairs in the doctor's stark office. Before her bottom had touched her chair she was talking about a growth, a mass, a tumour and treatment.

It wasn't real, they were all talking about Lucy but it couldn't be real. The doctor was adamant that Lucy should start chemotherapy although the final biopsy report, she said, was not ready.

Hadn't those reports shown that there were no problems? My brain faltered, I couldn't find the words to form the questions I wanted to ask. All I knew was that I couldn't leave Lucy in this woman's hands.

I was struggling, overcome once again with a sinking feeling.

Lucy's surgeon suggested waiting. She mentioned a second cancer clinic in the hospital and I found myself nodding to his suggestion to wait for the full biopsy report and check out the other clinic.

I was numb. Lucy and cancer didn't go together. That didn't fit in my brain, not at all, not after the wonderful feeling, the elation of getting through the operation and hearing that the test results were negative.

The meeting was over. Walking back towards 676, Maria and I talked briefly about her brother and my soon to be ex-husband.

'Yorgos needs to be here', Maria said. I nodded.

'Of course. He needs to know exactly what is happening to Lucy. Let me clear my head and I'll call him.'

'No', she said. 'I'll do that. We'll arrange for him to get a flight as soon as he can leave Rhodes.'

Maria and George left with Dr Dolatza and I returned to the hard chair at Lucy's bedside. I was dazed and Lucy was dazzling, chatting and laughing with little Eleni, who was suffering from an undiagnosed stomach disorder. Her pretty young mother had told me about what her bright two-year-old daughter had been through, the tests and hospital visits, and I had felt so sorry for them. This evening I saw shock and fear on Elpida's face.

I couldn't come to terms with the fact that in a matter of days, hours, minutes, with just a line from that doctor, our lives had changed. Lucy and I were going in a direction that I hadn't considered.

Who in their right mind would have thought that the laughing, cheeky child of so few days ago could be a cancer victim?

It's later, the room is in semi-darkness and everyone, including Lucy, is asleep. I am scribbling in a small exercise book I bought so I can keep a track of our days here and also, hopefully, so I can put words to some of my feelings and thoughts.

I dozed at some stage but don't know how. Lucy and I are still sharing the bed but she is not at all happy to have me as a bed partner. I have no choice. I can't sleep sitting upright on the chair that is tucked under her bed and it is way too cold to lie on the floor.

Lucy is on an antibiotic drip and I am scared of hurting her. I huddle, lying cramped against the window. The bed is next to a radiator, which was on full blast all night. I am either baking hot or freezing cold.

3

Sunday 9 December

Lucy has been in hospital for two weeks. I wonder if she will ever get out.

I must look a sight. I'm stiff and tired and can almost feel the dark shadows under my eyes, reminders of another sleepless night, watching Lucy's deep sleep.

Looking out the window I can see snow, like icing sugar, on the nearby Imitos hills. Hopefully that will be a good start for Lucy today.

I was right. Lucy woke with a smile, she was bright and apparently in no pain. Her smile was even broader when I told her that her father would be flying to Athens.

I spoke with many of my friends and my mobile hardly stopped ringing all day. Talking, however, was difficult and I found myself lost for words. 'Cancer' was enough, a conversation stopper.

Maria told me more about the operation although there were no official results. Cancerous cells were found among the neck glands that were removed and the doctors were talking of a type of cancer rarely found in children. She told me to put on a front, as if nothing too serious was happening.

'Be wary of what you say or do in front of or near Lucy. You can't break down.'

That's not going to be easy, Maria. Your niece is anything but stupid.

Leaving Lucy chatting to Elpida and Eleni, my brother-in-law, George, and I made our way down to the hospital's first floor to meet with cancer specialists in the other clinic. The Haematological and Oncology Unit (TAO in Greek) looked like any other ward as we pushed open a heavy red swing door and entered a warm and quiet clinic. I felt awful, a visitor in the wrong place. There were children moving about; one little boy (or girl) scooted past me, leaving the double doors to rock shut. The youngsters were like any other children except that they were all bald and most were connected to drips, the bottled medication hanging, jangling from mobile frames, with a computer-like machine in the middle.

'I can't bring Lucy down here. She'll freak when she sees these children. She'll know straight away that something's not right.'

I thought of her reaction when we had entered the overcrowded room on our first day in Agia Sofia. She'd been quick to remark on a pale little girl wearing a tight knitted hat, even though the room was unusually warm.

'Poor thing, she must have cancer, eh Mum? Isn't that what they wear Mum when kids have cancer?'

I told her to stop staring.

'I'm not staring,' she said, but she had looked away, as sad as the little face she had been watching.

George touched my arm, steering me through more swing doors to tap on the closed door on our right. I took a deep breath as we were ushered into the main office of the TAO clinic.

I froze and started to shake. I didn't expect the kind, sympathetic face I found myself looking at. Vasilis Papadakis, one of the TAO doctors, introduced himself. Late thirties, glasses outlining bright eyes, a likeable face framed by a light beard, he was wearing semi-casual baggy corduroys and a checked shirt. He looked more like a teacher than a cancer specialist, a far cry from the green-gowned director of the other clinic.

We talked about Lucy and her problem.

'It's probably a tumour,' he said, 'a malignant tumour with other cancerous cells that have spread to the glands.' He urged against immediate therapy, preferring to wait for other test results. 'I want to know exactly what we are dealing with,' he said.

I was shaking noticeably and saw the doctor take a deep breath. 'You must find the strength to get through this without showing your feelings, your anguish and your sorrow.'

I heard myself sigh. How? That seemed an impossible task.

Lucy had always managed to read my thoughts. Could I become an actress? What's Lucy going to be like? What will she go through?

Despite the questions, I knew that Lucy would be in good hands. I felt that we had made the right choice in finding an alternative clinic. We agreed to move Lucy into TAO as soon as possible.

I told Lucy we would be moving again. Surprisingly, she wasn't too worried. She quickly told Elpida and Eleni that she would keep in touch. We moved, not into the TAO clinic as there were no spare beds, but to another ward on the fourth floor. We were in a large, airy room with four beds, pullout divans and a large veranda.

This afternoon Yorgos arrived from Rhodes. Pale, concerned and visibly shaken, he seemed to be coping with all that his sister had told him. Lucy, of course, was over the moon, delighted to see him, and immediately stopped saying that she wanted to go home. In the evening Yorgos and I took Lucy downstairs to the clinic to talk with Dr Papadakis, who quietly outlined her illness. 'Lucy, you have a problem, an illness that will require treatment. You won't get better straight away but it can be cured.'

He was careful in his approach and his use of words. Cancer was mentioned a couple of times but not when he was talking directly to Lucy. She remained very cool, civil but not friendly. She broke into tears the moment we left his office. I was lost for words and support. There were other people, women and children, in the corridor as we left the doctor and moved into the waiting room area. I heard voices but saw nothing beyond Lucy's pinched and frightened face.

Lucy didn't mention the other children in the clinic. She nestled in to her father's arm as we took the lift back up to the fourth floor. She's usually too quick to comment on anything out of the ordinary. But then, what is ordinary now? Is Lucy so frightened that the world around her doesn't register? How are we going to cope with all this?

I can hardly cope with it, how will Lucy manage?

How will we both?

Monday 10 December

Today was somehow an easier day for Lucy. That sounds absurd, incongruous in these surroundings, but she was happier, brighter. In a strange way she has already settled into her new environment, chatting with the other children in the ward and the nursing staff. She seemed to be taking things in her stride, and even had a school lesson with a teacher on the ward while I went to meet with her surgeon again.

I was upset and I told him I felt misled and ignored before and after Lucy's surgery. A pained expression passed over his face.

'I know. I'm sorry but sometimes it's just better that way. We all cope with our problems in different ways. You were already shattered when you arrived here from Rhodes. We had to give you time.'

He assured me that the doctors were already hard at work on Lucy's case. They were considering a rare type of cancer and looking at immediate treatment. I wanted to hear more details but a phone call from the surgery ward cut our meeting short. Dr Dolatza hurried out the door and I walked away from his office clinging to the hope that the more tests they did, the better our situation.

What if the test results were wrong? What if Lucy wasn't that ill? A miracle could happen couldn't it? Something just might snap us out of this nightmare …

I walked to the small Saint Sofia chapel in the hospital gardens, next to the busy coffee shops. The small chapel had a regular clientele; all hoping for an answer to prayers invariably focused on the young occupants of the hospital a few metres away.

What God can put children, my little girl, in such a vulnerable situation? Is there a God? Is this how he celebrates the birth of his son? We had been getting ready for Christmas; the boys were looking forward to decorating the house, the surprise and excitement of that special day. Lucy had talked about fixing a new tree with Yanni. She couldn't wait to get out of Rhodes hospital to do that.

Instead our world had been turned upside down.

I left the chapel and returned to the ward disappointed and lost.

— ⁓ —

I called my sister, Pat, in New Zealand, dialling and closing the number a couple of times, thinking it wasn't the right moment; I wasn't in the right frame of mind to talk. But when would I be? I let the third attempt ring and then heard Pat's anguish on the other end of the line.

'Click off,' she said. 'I'll call you straight back.' I hung up and she called back immediately.

'What will you do when we can't be near you?' she asked.

Although I had settled half the world away from my family, we had remained extremely close. We were rarely out of touch, speaking regularly; there were no secrets. I knew I couldn't speak to Mum from that corridor connection, and Pat understood. She promised to talk with my mother, my sister Judy and Jim, our brother.

I put the phone down and sobbed.

The surgical ward is warm, bright and well lit compared with other parts of the hospital. Today it was heartless, grey. I dried my tears, made a quick visit to the toilet to ensure there were no telltale signs of my feelings, and walked back to our room to find Lucy laughing with her father.

Thank God she can laugh. She is my Lucy when she laughs, all blonde curls and sparkling eyes.

I didn't want to intrude so I hurried downstairs to another payphone and called my friends on Rhodes.

American-born Sheila, who has lived in the Lindos village for more than 30 years, was her usual self, sympathetic and practical at the same time. 'Just continue being you,' she said. 'You're a fighter; I know you're strong.' Her words brought tears. I didn't want to cry, didn't want to show my weakness.

'I'm not strong. I'm lost. I can't even speak when I need to. This is all happening so fast. I'm way out of my depth here and I don't know why I am so useless!'

'You're tired, you're shocked,' she said. 'I know you will get Lucy through this.'

I wanted to believe her; I wanted to regain my confidence through her words and was (yet again) thankful for the anonymity of the telephone.

My other friends were kind and supportive; some told me to pray, to look to God and the saints, but I've never been very good at that. What is 'God help me'? Is it a prayer or a cry for help?

Later that evening Lucy was called for another test, a magnetic scan. She wanted her father to stay with her in the examination room but that wasn't possible because of the metal plate he has in his knee, the result of a motorbike accident years ago. She wasn't happy when I joined her but there was no other choice; she didn't want to be alone.

The procedure was much the same as for the CAT scan only it took longer and was a great deal noisier. I would never have imagined such banging and clanging would come from a hospital machine. Lucy lay still and quiet as requested, her co-operative attitude amazing the nursing staff and technicians and surprising her father and me. Back on the ward she was tired and slept early after clinging to her father before he left to spend the night with his sister.

Around 10pm the TAO clinic called for us to move again. I panicked, worried about waking Lucy and frightening her again. I left her sleeping and went downstairs to the clinic that, unlike the rest of the hospital already in semi-darkness, was bright and busy. Children and adults were in the waiting room and the young patients were calling from their rooms. There was a lot going on even thought it was late, but it didn't seem to matter. I expected to see Dr Papadakis but was greeted by a tall, attractive doctor who immediately agreed that we could stay on the fourth floor and move early in the morning.

'Good idea not to wake your daughter, but you must be down here early to keep the bed,' she warned.

Lucy hadn't moved. She was sound asleep and looked so peaceful, so normal. I pulled out the divan bed, checked her once again, wondered how nothing showed to indicate she was so ill, and lay down. However, the escape I sought through sleep was impossible. I got up and made my way back down to the clinic, clomping down the stairs with bags, cuddly toys and balloons hanging off my arm. I left the things on the bed in TAO and spoke briefly to a couple of young boys who were anxious to know who would be moving in.

'You're going to have my daughter for company in the morning,' I told them.

'Wow, a girl in here,' they laughed.

A chubby boy in the next bed turned his back to me. 'I don't get on with girls,' he mumbled. I sat on the side of his bed, looking at the sad curve of his back, and quickly described Lucy. 'She's cute, blonde.' I almost said full of life but stopped myself, gagging on the thought that maybe she wasn't anymore. 'She's got three brothers so she's used to boys, you'll like her. I hope you'll help her fit in,' I added as I left.

Lucy was still asleep, sound asleep and very still, like an angel. She wasn't in the middle of the night though, when she realised I had moved some of her things. Then she was angry, very, very angry.

Wednesday 12 December

I woke early, wondering if I had slept at all, and left Lucy to wake after 9am. Maria had suggested that the doctors might have started the chemotherapy without saying anything as Lucy was still on a drip, so I approached Dr Papadakis. He was busy but we had a quick word and he was reassuring.

No therapy has started.

'We won't start,' he said, 'until we have searched every possibility and know exactly what we are dealing with.'

We moved into TAO, to the large room with two Albanian boys, Neilson and Petros, and a little Athenian, Alexandros. The boys were waiting for Lucy and within minutes they were all chatting, swapping stickers and drawing.

Lucy's first comments were whispered. 'Mum, the boy sleeping opposite doesn't have any hair; neither does the one in the next bed.

Why would they cut their hair like that?'

Perhaps she hadn't noticed the children on her first visit to TAO. What had she noticed? Had she been too preoccupied with her own problem to notice the other children? I choked and didn't really answer her, but busied her and myself with our clothes and her toys.

Alexandros woke and boldly introduced himself. There was no holding him back. 'Hi, wow, nice hair, what's your name?'

'Loukia. Some people call me Lucy'.

'I'm going to call you Luce. Got any crayons so we can draw together?'

Lucy slid off the bed and straight into a new friendship. It struck me how good they looked together, around the same age, with the same cheeky style. Neilson, who had warned me that he didn't have a particularly good way with girls, was quickly won over by Lucy, although he remained reserved – much quieter than the bubbly Alexandros.

We were just getting settled when a large mannish woman strode into the room. Hands on hips, feet slightly apart, she surveyed the room and its young occupants, who were suddenly quiet. This blue-uniformed nurses' aide had quite a presence. She had the ability to freeze what was a happy atmosphere. She turned towards Lucy and me.

'You're moving.' Panic. I felt as if there was no air in the room.

'Where to?'

'Don't look so worried. We're off to a smaller, quieter room, so repack your things. And get rid of those balloons and toys,' she huffed. 'All they do is gather dust and that's not allowed here.'

Neither Lucy nor I said anything. We repacked toys, balloons and all, and rather reluctantly followed her down the corridor to the first room near the entrance into the ward. Our abrupt guide pointed to the first of two beds and left without another word, holding the door open for Dr Dolatza, Lucy's surgeon. He sat on the side of the bed and opened a sketchpad Lucy had used over the past few days. He flicked through the pages and stopped at a drawing of children and balloons.

'I like that, Lucy. I love art and see a lot of drawings and, you know what, you've got talent. Can you draw something for me?' Lucy smiled and nodded.

Dr Dolatza removed the dressing on the side of Lucy's neck and cut the stitches, chatting all the time about the importance of art, of imagination, of balloons. He and the nurses suggested Lucy have a shower and they left. Her mood had altered with changing rooms. She was angry, looking at me with cold, accusing eyes, but in the shower, under the running water, she calmed down.

My God she is so little, vulnerable, breakable.

Lucy relaxed and was even happier when her father appeared. I was dismissed; neither wanted me around so I checked with the doctors who told me that we had to be at another hospital early tomorrow morning for a major bone scan.

I left the hospital and went window-shopping around the local stores, walking, talking to friends from Rhodes on my phone and thinking that just a few weeks ago I had vowed never to own a mobile. I still hated the thing but today I realised that I would be even more lost and isolated without it.

I walked for a couple of hours, probably in circles, but that didn't matter. I was out of that hospital, anonymous, wandering through a suburb of one of Europe's busy capital cities.

The children's hospitals – the Agia Sofia, one of the largest children's hospitals in Europe, and the adjacent Aglaia Kyriakou, named after its benefactors – were, it seemed, just two of many hospitals and clinics in that suburb of sprawling colourless buildings, apartments, supermarkets, snack bars and shops.

I walked until I could walk no more and returned to TAO, to Lucy in that small room. We were sharing with a couple, Sofia and Yanni, and their daughter Marina, from Rhodes. They were not very talkative and I didn't like to ask what was wrong with Marina. I believe she was being treated for leukemia. Marina was 20 months old.

It's evening now and Lucy is asleep after a few hours in the small playroom they have here for the children in TAO. I hadn't noticed the room, which is at the end of the ward near the large dayroom. Alexandros invited Lucy to join him there and she fitted in perfectly.

Is that good or bad? I'd be happier if she didn't have to fit in, didn't have to stay.

I felt a horrible weight, an ache in my stomach, as I watched her listen carefully to the young girls who opened the playroom this afternoon. They welcomed all the children by name, chatted to Lucy, asking her what she liked to do and within minutes she was busy, learning to decorate a bottle by wrapping it with twine. She painted and, prompted by one of the young girl's guitar playing, sang along with the other children, their voices and music drifting throughout the clinic.

I'm happy that Lucy has new friends and company but there were a lot of questions today.

'Why don't these kids have any hair Mum?' I told her it must have something to do with their illness and that I was sure it would grow back. 'Really? Okay, strange though isn't it?'

Earlier I'd gone shopping with Maria, who bought some new clothes for her niece. I don't know how long we are going to be in Athens so I must be careful with money. The basic hospital charges will be covered by my national insurance healthcare, but will there be extras? I can't afford to be extravagant so I watched as Maria chose some lovely things for Lucy: new jackets, tops, a scarf and a cute hat and little gloves. We returned to TAO laden with shopping bags, all for Lucy, but she wasn't impressed, not interested at all.

She didn't even want to look at her other visitor, her grandfather Stamatis, who braved the clinic and its children, armed with presents and a big, cautious smile. I'd not met him before; he had separated from my mother-in-law 40 years ago, leaving her with two young children. Contact between father and son had remained minimal. A lightly built, quietly spoken and pleasant man, he was nothing like the ogre I'd imagined. I was pleasantly surprised.

As Stamatis left, Xenia introduced herself as a specialist in child psychology and originally from Lindos. I knew neither Xenia's background nor her qualifications but that didn't matter, she was the evening's bright note, flowing into the ward with an infectious laugh and a grin that brightened our surroundings.

It was nearly midnight when I called Pat again. Mum, she said, had sobbed while listening to her news, but she was adamant that Lucy would sparkle again and already had the whole of her residential care home, Nazareth House, praying for her grand-daughter's recovery.

I wonder if prayers can heal.

Why can't I find the faith that my Dutch friend and colleague Aty has, to believe that prayers will be answered?

Aty is sensible and can often see things in a way that I can't. I sought her help and support when Yorgos and I separated. Then, over endless cups of coffee and cigarettes, she told me to be strong; she was adamant that my life would improve. She gave me the same advice a few days ago. Be strong, pray. God and the Lord will hear you.

Will he?

Thursday 13 December

Lucy's name day. What a place to celebrate.

We were up early to go to Sotirias (Saviour) Hospital before 8am and Lucy's anger was at its best, wild when I had to get her out of bed and flaming when the vein in her hand collapsed as the nurse gave her an antibiotic. The bloodied butterfly clip was taken out and we hurried off.

Cuddled close to her father, Lucy sat quietly in the back seat of the Mercedes as her uncle inched our way through the early Athens traffic to reach the hospital a good 30 minutes before its nuclear medicine department opened. I wondered what nuclear medicine had to do with a bone scan, glaringly aware yet again of my total lack of knowledge of such things. Fortunately Lucy wasn't in the mood to ask questions, as I had no answers.

When the office did open the nurse abruptly told us to return quickly to Agia Sofia to renew the link into Lucy's vein. Panic. The nurse at Agia Sofia had been adamant that they would do it at Sotirias and now we were being sent back.

Lucy cried all the way. Cried, moaned and talked us through all the grisly details of those nurses in Rhodes making holes in her hands, hurting her.

'I want to go home. Please, I just want to go home.'

Her father tried to pacify her as his patient brother-in-law crawled through the ever-increasing traffic. I sat back, nursing a heavy stomach and aching heart.

What's happening to my little girl? She was so upset, so miserable, and we could do nothing to cheer her up.

We hurried back into TAO, had the intravenous needle and clip replaced and, against all odds and the unbelievable Athens traffic, returned quickly to Sotirias to be told that we would have to wait in a grubby staffroom at the back of the laboratory. The well-meaning staff wanted to isolate Lucy from the other (much older) outpatients to keep her away from germs. They were trying to protect her but I wondered if it was too late.

At midday the head doctor, a strange but gentle man that Yorgos didn't like and I felt immediately drawn to, gave Lucy an injection and explained that we had to sit for another two hours to allow the dye to run through her veins. The test, he said, would run later in the afternoon. I left Lucy with her father and I wandered off to find the hospital canteen. Heavy rain put an end to any thought of venturing outside, so I returned to the staffroom and found Lucy asleep in her father's arms.

He's very good with her, loving and caring, maybe too soft at times, I thought. But where is that man I adored? Maybe I am not trying hard enough, but I can't see him anymore.

The hours passed slowly, without small talk. Yorgos and I had nothing in common save our unspoken thoughts about Lucy and, later, our relief when the doctor assured us that the test was clear.

'I understand your anxiety,' he said, 'so I have checked the results quicker than usual. This is one test you don't have to worry about; there are no signs of cancer in your daughter's bones.'

Good news. I felt almost elated, but my high spirits weren't to last. Lucy returned to Agia Sofia with her father and I went to my in-laws to shower, eat and to try to relax. They did their best to chat, to lighten things, but the atmosphere was uncomfortable and there was a heavy feeling of doom pervading the room. After dinner we sat talking by Maria's fireplace, sharing a rare cigarette and a glass of wine. There was so much to discuss but little was said; we were all stuck in our own thoughts and the usually soothing flame of the open fire did little to warm our spirits and conversation.

My mobile buzzed and it was Xenia. She said she had spoken with Lucy's specialist and treatment would start tomorrow and last around eight months.

Eight months.

I was numb, taking in the words, trying to imagine what Lucy was going to go through. Perhaps if I could learn more about this cancer, Lucy's enemy, where it was and what it was like, then I would be more confident with the doctors and our surroundings.

I returned to the hospital later than planned and Lucy was angry, bitter and wild. Sometimes I feel that she can't stand to be near me and can't stand for me to be away from her. Yorgos' influence on her emotional and psychological state could be more positive, but maybe I am being unfair. Guess she has to take out her anger and fear on something or someone and that someone is going to be me.

I went shopping for Lucy's name day, buying cakes and gifts, anything to make her feel better, but there were too many people around her this evening. They were well meaning, wanting to cheer her up, but Lucy was grumpy and she didn't want to look at them, let alone speak to them.

Later in the evening her doctor was on call. He sat on the edge of Lucy's bed and explained that she would start therapy in the morning. But first she had to return to surgery.

Lucy's eyes flashed, brimming with tears. 'Surgery again?' Her fear was silent, palpable and painful. He took her hand and looked straight into her eyes.

'Don't worry Lucy. We are going to give you a plug, a Hickman line it is called. It won't hurt and you will never have to worry about needles and painful jabs again. Okay? I promise you, this will help you get better. Trust me.'

I asked if we could talk alone and treated him to one of Lucy's name day cakes.

He explained the situation. 'Lucy's tumour is malignant and dangerous. Surgery is out of the question because of its position but a combination of chemotherapy and radiation treatment hopefully will stop it. The treatment should take about eight months. There is,' he said, 'no guarantee.'

I asked about the Hickman and he described it as a silicon catheter, a special intravenous line into a vein near the heart.

'It's used for giving fluids and medication and also for taking blood samples so Lucy won't have to put up with the needle pricks she hates. It's minor surgery,' he said, explaining that part of the catheter would be tunnelled under the skin of her chest, the tip resting in a large vein just above the heart and coming out from a small cut in her chest where there would be a couple of stitches. 'I know it sounds complicated but it will make Lucy's life much easier at the moment. She will just have to be careful.'

He took a deep breath.

'This isn't going to be easy, not for Lucy, not for you, not for us. Her treatment is going to be difficult, harsh, and Lucy will have problems with her mouth and gums. This tumour,' he explained, 'is like a floating mass, somewhere between her nose and throat. It's in an area we use every day to eat, to breathe. Lucy is going to have to be extra careful to stay clear of infections; a simple cold could be catastrophic. She must stay away from germs.'

We talked about schooling. Lucy would not be able to go to school but there was a teacher available in the clinic in the mornings. I felt it would be important to keep the thread of lessons, of normality. Everything must be as it was and will be whenever we are back in Rhodes. Lucy will go back to her school.

A telephone call put an end to our conversation and I left the doctor and found myself thinking of the boys.

How would they feel when they heard about their little sister?

How would they react? How would they cope?

Phew.

I would have to sit down and talk with Yorgos. We'd been separated for nearly a year so if I was going to be in Athens for months we would have to decide where the boys would live, what would happen with their schooling, their extra lessons. Heavens, Yanni would be sitting national exams at the end of the school year. I was starting to feel panicky again when Xenia appeared. A godsend, so quiet, kind and unassuming in her layers of nondescript clothing and comfortable shoes. Xenia wouldn't stand out in a crowd but she is one very special lady. She has the smile and the eyes of a ray of sunshine. We talked, a lot, and it was late by the time she left. Even though it had been a full day I wasn't at all tired.

I called Judy in Australia and turned quickly to my notebook afterwards.

God, how I miss my family, my friends. Talking to Jude makes me realise just how alike we are. We used to be so different and yet our lives have run along parallel lines. Jude's ten years older than me, the family rebel who left home at 16 and was always out with a boyfriend that Dad never knew about. At 19 Jude was married with a child and at 20 she was telling doctors there was something wrong with her little girl, explaining that Tania suffered fits, convulsions. The doctors tested the nine-month-old baby and suggested that my sister see a specialist, preferably a psychologist. They said the fits were a figment of her imagination.

They were wrong. A few months later another doctor found a brain tumour. Four-year-old Tania died in 1969.

By then Judy had a second daughter, Keri, and later a son, Gavin. In the early 1980s, when I left London to live on Rhodes, my sister, her husband and young family moved to Australia to settle in Melbourne. It was a new life but the memory of Tania remained as the marriage failed and Jude's life took another road.

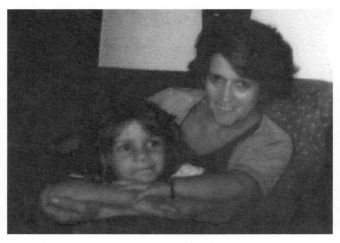

At home: my sister Jude had called me during the summer after seeing this photo. She'd said how alike we were: 'We have the same hurting eyes.' I'd laughed but her words echoed as I considered our failed marriages and daughters with cancer

Jude called me during the summer after seeing a photo of Lucy and me taken in my sitting room. I thought it was a good mother and daughter photo, warm and loving.

Jude commented on how alike we were. We have the same hurting eyes, she said.

I had laughed at her words but they haunt me now as I consider our failed marriages and daughters with cancer.

Friday 14 December

It's 10.45am and Lucy's back from surgery. She's asleep; she looks shattered and has a Hickman plug.

Please God let us get through this. It's not fair, it's not right, to put such a gorgeous innocent little girl through this.

Whose fault is it? Should I have been more cautious, quicker to take her to other doctors?

Is the cancer from something I wasn't careful about?

Am I to blame?

The same questions run through my head all day, every day. I can't stop thinking, wondering how this can be happening to my daughter.

I fear I am going to go mad.

I've lost weight and must look drained. Xenia suggested I buy some vitamins. At just over 50 kgs I have to be careful or I'll end up looking like the witch that Lucy often calls me ...

Lucy started her first dose of chemotherapy, the drugs dripping into her body via the Hickman plug. She is now one of those children I saw and pitied when I first came to TAO, a tiny child wired to a moveable frame. She is on an intravenous drip and the nurses syringe her drugs into the tubes. I then 'rinse' them through the drip system. Ah, it looked easy, but when they asked me to do it, I was all thumbs, twisting the bottles and squeezing tubes with shaking hands.

Nothing happened.

The nurses repeated the procedure and all was well. I tried and the drip stopped, the whole thing filling with the drug. The nurses took over once again.

I suspect they think I'm an idiot.

Hooked up to her medication, Lucy dozed most of the day and Yorgos and I met with the clinic director, Dr Haidas. He described the tumour as a 'nasopharyngeal carcinoma, undifferentiated, non-keratinised.'

They were just words, medical terms, and a title for Lucy's illness. I didn't understand them but wrote them down anyway, determined to learn about them at some stage.

The cancer, Dr Haidas said, could be treated with chemotherapy and radiotherapy, treatment that would take about eight months. That much I knew already.

Haidas, a short, stocky man with no outstanding characteristics save larger than normal ears, put Lucy's chances of a normal life at 50–50.

I spoke to Lucy's surgeon, who accepted cakes for Lucy's name day and gave her one of his own small watercolours. We talked about art. Dr Dolatza sketched and painted, had had works exhibited and also wrote – not just medical books but children's books, which he illustrated. I appreciated his gift, it was special, a nice touch for Lucy. I felt that he would be a good contact in that hospital.

My brother-in-law picked me up mid-afternoon and I went to eat and shower at my in-laws, a change, and a temporary escape from the hospital.

Their bathroom is my haven. I can hide my feelings all day but as soon as I lock the door, head for that cold tub, the tears fall, uncontrolled. I cry and sob under the shower and into the towel so no one can hear me. I cry for my little girl who is hurting, I cry until the water cools and then I dry off, dress, take a deep breath and unlock the door.

The tears stop with the click of that key.

I return to the real world, outwardly calm and collected, and later in the evening, back to TAO.

Lucy must have a daily shower, which is nothing new, but the performance of getting her showered is. First I have to get Lucy, myself, and her frame into the small shower cubicle opposite our room. Then there's the struggle to get her undressed, ensuring that the drip is functioning, the

Hickman line isn't tangled and Lucy isn't getting angry. I have to wash her thoroughly, without getting the Hickman dressing wet. I'm edgy, wary of hurting her and damaging the line.

After tonight's shower Lucy was cold and shivery but refused to put on pyjamas, preferring her nightgown. If she rejects something, that's it, she's stubborn, unusually strong and determined, and she doesn't back down.

This evening I cleaned and changed the dressing on the Hickman. I had help from one of the nurses and guidance from Sophia but still my hands shook as I tried to put on the sterilised gloves without touching everything in sight. Off came the patch, and then I did the cleaning. I made a coil out of the small plastic pipe that seems to have become part of Lucy's chest, covered it with a new dressing, sticky tape, and, that was it. Finished.

Lucy looked like she was ready to spit at me. I bent to give her a kiss but she was too quick. She turned and left me staring at her back.

God, how am I going to do this? My first aid skills are basic and I feel cumbersome, useless and ignorant.

It's after 10 and this place is extremely busy, people and kids everywhere. It's late in the evening that the clinic seems to come alive, doors that are closed all day are thrown open, the children mingle and parents chat in the corridor, in the waiting room and out in the entrance area. No one makes any attempt to get the children into bed early.

Strange.

But on second thought I guess it makes sense. What would you get them into bed early for? What do they have to look forward to after a good night's sleep?

What can you promise them?

Not a lot.

Saturday 15 December

This morning I woke early after an awful night following Lucy's first taste of chemotherapy. She had a high temperature, was very restless during the few hours she managed to sleep and seemed to wake to pee every hour. Getting Lucy to and from the toilet was a complicated procedure, becoming worse the more tired we became.

On her 'Mum' I had to move quickly, get her out of bed, helping her and the frame out of the room and across the corridor and into the bathroom. The frame, with its bottles and the computer-like machine that was programmed to suit each child's medication, wouldn't slide properly. Pulling and lifting it, I had to guide Lucy, ensuring that the tubes connected to her Hickman weren't twisted, couldn't catch on the frame and, at the same time, watch that I didn't pull them too tight or too far away from her body. Twice I forgot that the machine was plugged in to the wall to recharge above her bed. We hurried off, only to be jolted back by the lines.

God, what a performance! No doubt it would have been funny to watch were we in other, not so heartbreaking, circumstances.

Yorgos was in the clinic early.

It's strange to have him in my life again. We've been through so much together and I guess something like Lucy's illness could bring us back together.

I doubt it though.

Lucy woke angry. She didn't want to get dressed, really didn't want to do anything. She had vomited during the night and continued heaving, the sickness racking her little body. It was distressing and quite frightening but the nurses told me not to worry, that it was a normal reaction to this therapy. The doctor coaxed her into conversation and Lucy joined the other children in the TAO waiting room. Volunteers from a local charity were organising a Christmas workshop. The children were reserved, at first reluctant to make the decorations demonstrated by the volunteers. It was quiet and withdrawn Neilson who succeeded in getting everyone involved. He surprised us all, including himself, when the paper he was cutting turned into a sparkling Christmas star. Delight lit up his face, treating us to a glimpse of the happy boy he once was, and encouraging the other children, including Lucy, to take part. Within minutes tassels, coloured paper and tinsel filled the air and every corner of the room.

The waiting room looked a different, warmer place afterwards.

Little Marina and her parents left today. As soon as they left I opened the window and the curtains billowed as cool, fresh air filled the small room. The fresh air was not to last. The nurses were still changing the bed and the cot when Panayiota moved in and her mother promptly shut the window.

Panayiota is 14 and is another leukemia patient. She's a big, cumbersome girl, her short hair in tight curls framing a round, freckled face. Her smile is sad, reserved, and she has awful stretch marks on her arms. As I write this she is tucking in to crisps and croissants, the empty packets folding noisily into the sheets as she moves restlessly on her bed. She wears a surgical mask most of the time and her mother Maria is very protective, overprotective even. If her looks could kill, anyone coming to see Lucy would be dead. She keeps saying that her daughter has a temperature and that her white blood cell level is far too low, but that means little to me.

What I do understand is her worried face and blunt, stressed speech.

Sunday 16 December

I woke worn-out and aching after a difficult, sleepless night.

Poor Lucy. She was restless again, plagued by a high temperature, vomiting and, every hour on the hour, wanting to pee.

The nurses had introduced a new system to get us through the night. Instead of running to the toilet opposite, Lucy peed into a bottle. I don't know which is more difficult, getting her out of bed and across the corridor to the toilet or having her pee into the cut-off plastic water bottle. I measured the urine and wrote it all down as what comes out of her body has to be monitored equally as much as what is going into her system, then I washed it down the toilet.

I'm tired and depressed, everything seems black, an unmanageable near future. Seems like sickness and despair is all around us and any strength or optimism I felt over the past few days has disappeared.

I went for a walk, but constant drizzle kept me relatively close to the hospital and the grey overcast sky did nothing to lift my spirits. What did help were calls from my close friends, Sharon and Gro.

They were my lifesavers today. I had walked out of the Agia Sofia gate with my head down, full of negative thoughts, and returned feeling positive.

Lucy will get better.

It was a day of waiting. Waiting for the nurses, waiting for my sister-in-law to arrive. Waiting for what? A change? A miracle?

When I wasn't thinking about Lucy my thoughts were on the boys. I hoped and prayed that they wouldn't be affected too much by Lucy's illness and my absence. Lucy could annoy the hell out of them at times but usually they were good company together. The boys were proud and protective of their little sister, they loved her.

At home they were used to having their grandmother in the house. My worry was not so much about during the day; it was more during the evening hours when the twins, especially, could be a handful. Yanni would manage; he knew how to fill his hours and to choose his friends. Fit, good looking, he was an easy mixer with the ability

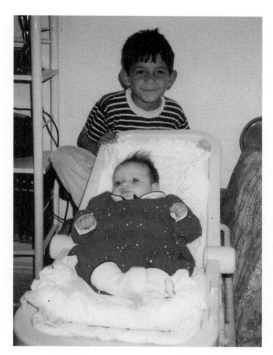

Lucy with her proud older brother Sam
(Stamatis in Greek)

to be good at whatever he tried. The twins were another story. Good humoured, funny and adventurers, they revelled in a totally different approach: they were not so focused. As toddlers they were always good company for one another, getting each other in and out of mischief. They remained affectionate, huggers who more often than not sat on or over one another, legs entwined, to watch television, the reflecting mirror balance of twins.

They were brothers and best friends but they were also 14, volatile and hot blooded and, if provoked, fought like adults. They didn't just use the cursing bad language of older men; Tony and Sam brawled, punched and boxed.

However, it was the company they would seek after school and during the weekends that worried me. I'd always been careful to get them involved in sports and activities after school. Like Yanni they had tried athletics, swimming and kayaking. I was with them at national

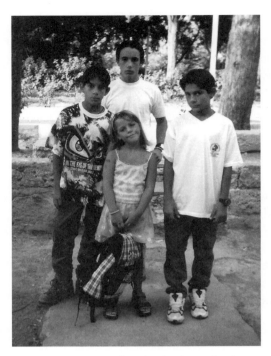

In the yard, the first day back to school
after summer holidays

championships when they managed to argue in a two-man kayak, an angry tangle of arms and paddles until they found their rhythm to continue on and finish the race. They weren't so interested in sports but did enjoy art lessons and, more recently, had started to learn how to play classical guitar. They were gifted with an ear for music, according to their teacher. She and I had laughed at the contrast, fine classical tunes juxtaposed against the twins' rather extreme images of spiked hair, huge baggy jeans falling off their backsides over thin thighs, sagging on to over-sized shoes. The guitar lessons would keep them busy for a while but what of all the other hours when I knew they would seek the company and cheek of other rougher Old Town boys?

How can I check them from here? Will their grandmother be able to maintain control? Will their father take any notice?

Maybe I was worrying for nothing.

Time would tell.

It's late and Lucy is going through an extremely difficult time. She's been sick many times, the vomiting matched by a burning, vicious anger.

How would I feel watching these drugs dripping in to my body?

Would I have the same feelings and reactions?

Monday 17 December

Lucy looked better this morning. She was vomiting less and her temperature was near normal. However, another side effect of her strong medication was noticeable: she was starting to lose her hair. There were wispy strands everywhere, on her pillow, her clothes, and clogging the hairbrush. I didn't say anything to Lucy and she was too sick to notice.

Yorgos was in TAO early again, just in the door as Panayiota was called for surgery to have another Hickman put in. I had thought Panayiota was in TAO for a check-up but I was wrong. Would she have to start treatment all over again? I didn't know and it was not the right time to ask.

It was a quiet morning, mainly because we could hardly speak to Lucy. She was hostile, particularly angry with me whenever her father was in the room. She didn't want to do anything, refused to lie on her bed and was curled up asleep on the chair when her doctor arrived.

'Don't worry, just let her be,' he said. Phew, was she mad, unusually annoyed with Dr Papadakis and vicious with me. It hurt to see her like that. Her anger was raw, close to hatred.

Tuesday 18 December

It's very early, not even 7am. Lucy and all the other children on TAO are still asleep and I'm drinking my first coffee. I was up before the lights went on in the ward and I crept into the communal showers that we, the parents, aren't meant to use. I was in and out of there before the ward started to come to life, a quick, almost guilty, shower under the hot water before anyone could catch me. Crazy but I do feel better, cleaner, and more human!

Lucy's father and her aunt are adamant that we show the biopsy results to other doctors. They are right to want a second opinion but I am so confident with these doctors that I feel awkward broaching the subject with Lucy's specialist. Stupid me.

Chris has already contacted a Harley Street specialist in London who is interested in Lucy's case. I just have to get up the courage to ask for all the details and send them on to him.

Panayiota and Lucy have struck up a friendship, despite their age difference. They chat, talk themselves to sleep, and wake and chat again. Panayiota, a big lump of a girl, was telling Lucy about her life.

'Ah, Lucy,' she said, 'I didn't always look like this. My hair was longer than yours; I was thinner and pretty, just like all the other girls. Now I can't look in a mirror, guess I don't need to look in a mirror to see the monster I've become. Look at my arms, Lucy! They shouldn't look like that. I know it is the cortisone that has blown me up, stretched me like a balloon. I hope you won't have to take it. But what am I saying, you're not ill.

'You're so young and healthy there is no way you can understand what I have gone through here.'

She talked about her medication and her long stay in isolation in the bone marrow transplant unit on the hospital's fourth floor.

'My sister was my donor, isn't that something? She's younger than I am but has already given me part of her life.'

She talked and talked until her eyes glazed with bitter tears and she was suddenly silent, slipping back into her world, somewhere only Panayiota could go. A tiny Lucy noticed the change and carefully turned to face Panayiota.

'Ah, come on Panayiota,' she said. 'Don't be like that. Give us a smile; you are so pretty when you smile. Here, catch mine ...'

Lucy smiled and Panayiota's pained expression changed as she gazed across the beds at Lucy. She sighed.

'Okay, Lucy. Throw me a smile!'

Lucy did and Panayiota's face lit up.

The two girls grinned and a deep friendship was born. It was as if they had known each other for years. I watched their faces and understood that Panayiota felt and hurt for Lucy. The poor teenager had been through it all. How was it that I saw the same look on Lucy's face?

~

Panayiota's mum, Maria, was separated and on her own with two other children. We talked. She gave me advice on how to cope on the ward and then introduced us to her collection of icons; icons and saints that she believed would help her daughter.

I tried to pay attention as she spoke, hoping I could learn something from her saints, but I found myself more aware of Maria than her words. She'd been overpowering and blunt when they had arrived but I realised that she was simply worried out of her mind about her daughter. As she introduced us to the painted icons that were tucked away under Panayiota's pillow, Maria's features changed dramatically. She softened; the tone of her voice dropped as she whispered the saints' stories and explained how they could help her daughter.

Pushing her dark hair back from her eyes she started with the Virgin Mary. 'She is the Ultimate Mother. She cares for every child, her love and concern has no boundaries.' Maria's touch on the icon was a caress and she kissed it lightly. 'This is Saint Antonios. He gave everything he had to the poor, he was a wise listener and everyone flocked to him for advice. This is Saint Savas, full of grace and truth and here are the saints Raphael, Nicholas and Irene, shown together on an icon from Lesbos. You must have heard of it. Their story is very famous,' she said, and then continued in a whisper that held Lucy and I mesmerised. 'Saint Raphael was the abbot of Karves, near the village of Thermi on the Greek island of Lesbos. Saint Nicholas was a deacon at the monastery and Saint Irene was the 12-year-old daughter of the mayor of Thermi. The three saints were at the monastery when Turkish invaders raided it. They were tortured and killed and remained unknown for many years, 500 or more. But you know what, Lucy? In 1959 the three saints appeared to the local people in dreams and visions. They guided excavations of their own grave, called people to repentance and cured all sorts of diseases. I know they will help Panayiota.'

As Maria explained her icons I realised that they weren't just religious drawings, like little medals to keep you safe; to her they were very real, a vital part of her life and possibly a huge part of her strength.

Thursday 20 December

I haven't written for a couple of days and don't really know why. Sitting and writing usually relaxes me and helps sort my thoughts. Maybe it's because we have settled into a routine and it feels like nothing new has happened.

God help us.

Lucy continues her first treatment. The bottles empty and are replaced, the drugs dripping into her little body. The nurses showed me how to flush or rinse the tubes, check the machine, and watch that the Hickman line wasn't pulled or twisted. Now I wonder what else I will have to learn.

Lucy was sick several times during the night and she has stopped eating. Despite Dr Papadakis' assurance that she is getting all the vitamins and fluids she needs, I continue to worry. She has a very sore nose; it's like herpes has invaded her nostrils and I fear it is one of those things we are going to have to get used to, to be careful about.

The mornings are particularly trying. Lucy is extremely difficult, touchy and angry, and doesn't want to dress. Once I manage to get her up she's fine. By then, however, I am shattered and my nerves are blown. Lucy is as normal as she can be here, bright and chatty with everyone. I want to crawl into a corner and cry.

I can't so I don't.

The Archbishop of Greece and Athens, Father Christodoulos, made a pre-Christmas visit to the children in TAO today. It was quite a performance, pre-empted by an earlier show from Eleni, the domineering nurses' aide who had moved us on our first day on TAO.

She made sure everything was clean and ready, and just after midday had all the children back in their rooms, sitting calmly on their beds. Parents with untidy bedside cabinets were ticked off as Eleni, lips pressed tightly together, strode through the ward, turning her head slowly from side to side, her eyes narrowing to spot anything she had missed. Nothing on her ward was going to be out of place.

There was commotion in the usually empty hospital entrance where plush red carpet had been hurriedly rolled down the steps. Television channels were there to capture the Archbishop spreading his Christmas cheer and to show everyone in Greece that they had a caring man at the head of their church.

I felt he could have visited the ward without the fanfare.

Father Christodoulos was used to the spotlight; he knew how to work it, flowing through the swinging doors of the TAO right on cue and turning left into our room to greet Lucy. He had a big smile, the kind smile and twinkling eyes of a Father Christmas when Santa figures really were caring old men. I didn't like all the fuss but had to admit that there was something very special about this man, an aura, charisma, and a quality that set him apart from others in the Greek Orthodox hierarchy. He blessed Lucy and surprised her with a big doll in a box, and left Panayiota with an electric organ.

It was all rather overpowering; one minute he was in the room and the next he was gone, his flowing gowns and entourage moving further into the ward.

An eerie silence followed. Both girls were overwhelmed with the whole performance. Lucy was sitting rather awkwardly on her bed, the huge, boxed doll across her legs. She turned the box towards her, bemused and not altogether happy. The battery-operated, walking talking doll was rather old fashioned, ungainly and strikingly similar to one I had dreamt of owning as a child.

In TAO this doll was too big, a bit too grand. Lucy would have preferred a Barbie. The girls were funny together, though. Lucy quickly had the doll frog-marching across the room as Panayiota mastered the basics of the organ. They played music, sang carols and giggled, forgetting their illnesses until they were warned by Eleni to be quieter. The organ was put back in its box and stored under the bed, and the carols and the laughter were short lived.

Life was a bitch in TAO.

Over the past few days we have gotten to know other children, and their parents, on the ward. Alexandros remains our favourite. The dazzling little boy who welcomed Lucy on her first day, is, as I suspected, another leukemia patient. He's extraordinary, bounding into the room and bouncing on Lucy's bed as if he's enjoying a pyjama party. With his cheeky grin and laughing dark eyes, he's a little rascal who would be into any mischief were he not in this cancer clinic. He's that type of a child; he oozes life and possesses a self-assurance that I've not seen in any other child in TAO. It's like this is his world and he has welcomed Lucy into it without restraints, without limits. Alexandros is one of the few who can easily break Lucy's moods. He makes her smile and won't take no for an answer. His mother, Joanna, is a tall, good-looking woman who carries herself well and is always well groomed, with the style of a wealthy French business woman. She's confident and strong but I wonder if her rather defiant throw-back the hair look hides her pain and worry.

Katerina, I imagine, is Lucy's age, and has leukemia. I don't know why but she has been in intensive care and is in a wheelchair with her parents Eleni and Spiros constantly at her side. They're a quiet, unassuming couple, who have eyes only for their daughter's needs.

There's another very thin boy, dark skinned with eyes as black as his hair, who is with his grandfather. There is a baby with leukemia whose mum is a young gypsy girl of 18. Yanni is a gangly, thin boy in his early teens who is with his parents, and then another pale little boy, Dimitri, who rarely ventures out of his room.

Those children who are able to get out of bed tend to get together around 3pm. The girls from The Smile of the Child Foundation arrive in TAO at about that time. Those young women, some volunteers, others employed by the charity, are a breath of fresh air as they breeze through the ward, pied pipers gathering children as they move towards the small playroom that quickly transforms into an area of laughter, sunshine and activity. The children forget they are ill and wired to medication stands, they become friends and find love and support in one another.

Joanna, a stunning girl with a wide smile and deep brown eyes, her dark hair held off her face by a thick band, told me about The Smile of the Child.

'The association was created by a ten-year-old boy in 1995. Our young founder's name was Andreas, and he suffered from terminal cancer. He was a rather shy, reserved boy, blonde with blue eyes and a big smile, who loved basketball and dancing. He also kept a diary.

'On 9 November 1995, Andreas wrote about setting up a foundation that would help the street children he would see from his carseat on the way to and from the hospital. His entry read: "We all know and talk about children in the streets who can't smile. They can't smile because they don't have money, or toys, or food and some of them don't even have parents. Just think and leave all the talking behind, let's unite and give whatever we can to poor children, Albanians, white and black. They are all children and deserve a smile. This association will be called The Smile of the Child. Let's help; if we unite we can accomplish it.'"

Joanna smiled as she spoke about Andreas' father establishing the charity. 'It's an amazing team, one that fights to protect children's rights, to provide emotional and psychological support, and, as you can see, to help children who are suffering from health problems,' she said. She left me a copy of the charity's newsletter and returned to help her young charges with their puzzles and paintings. 'When a child's smile fades, the whole world darkens.' The charity's slogan was powerful, as was the feeling that Joanna and her playroom colleagues sparked throughout TAO.

In the TAO playroom: Lucy never missed a chance to join in the singing, coaxed on by the multi-talented Joanna from The Smile of the Child

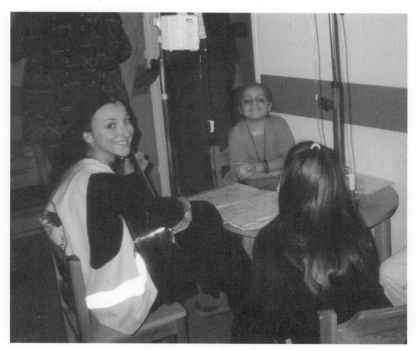

I wonder that the parents couldn't use such a playroom as well.

We meet in the corridors, in the waiting room, outside on the steps of the hospital, an area that is something of an open-air cafeteria, the TAO smoking lounge. I rarely smoke now but there are a lot of mums and dads who do. I join them for coffee and chats, and it's a get to know one another area, where stories are told, secrets and fears are shared; a psychologist's couch without the specialist and nothing but cold marble steps to sit on. That doesn't matter, nor does the cold, damp weather. It's the support, the understanding and the feelings shared that count.

As a newcomer I feel a bit of an outsider to this group. I listen as they talk of low blood counts, blood tests and new therapies. I'm an eavesdropper to conversations over cups of coffee that rarely empty. Whoever runs off to the hospital canteen or kiosk always returns with extra coffees, another pack of cigarettes.

Maria pulled me into the circle. 'Colleen, this is part of TAO and you will thank God that you have this companionship.' With a deep sigh she'd looked right into my eyes, somehow touching my thoughts and my fears. 'It's like a club that you would rather not join. But like it or not you become a member, you become part of the TAO family and it's these moments, the hospital step conversations and revelations, that sometimes keep you sane.'

Maria talked about her other children, her ex-husband, and her fears of Panayiota having to start therapy again. Joanna provides lighter conversation and Thanasis, in TAO at his son's bedside and one of the few fathers here without his wife's company as she is caring for a new baby, worries about his family's finances.

Everyone on those TAO steps has their own tale to tell. We have one thing in common: a fight. We are in a war against cancer; we are battling to bring our children's good health back.

Martin, an old school friend from New Zealand, called today. How he'd heard about Lucy I was not quite sure.

'Colleen', he said, 'if you need anything just let me know. I'm sending you some money that might help. But call me if you need me'.

I do need you Martin, you and all of my friends. Not just for money. I feel desperate for your conversation and our ties with the past, with normality, the bond with a Colleen that has little in common with the present-day one.

Gro called again this evening, telling me she had met Sharon and Sheila at a Christmas carol service in Rhodes' Evangelismo waterfront cathedral. 'We've decided you guys need our help. We're going to have a Christmas bazaar for you and Lucy, mulled wine, cakes, whatever we can make or find to sell.' She wouldn't listen to my protests and clicked off leaving me to wonder how my three closest friends had found one another.

I was still holding my mobile when the door opened and the twins walked into our room, surprising not just me but also Lucy, who very nearly pulled her Hickman line out leaping up to greet them. Hugs, kisses, smiles, the feeling was so good, so intense. Yanni was behind them with his grandmother at his side and suddenly my family was breaking every visiting rule at TAO.

They took the place by storm, much to our roommates' dismay. In between the misty kisses and hugs I tried to get them to come in one at a time, but their enthusiasm, as always, was overwhelming. Lucy was delighted to see them one moment, wanted them all out the next. So they took turns and in between bedside chats with their sister sat in the TAO waiting room taking in their surroundings.

'Oh, Mum, this is pretty heavy, isn't it? What's going on? Lucy doesn't look much different but she must be the only girl in here. None of these boys even have any hair!' Tony whispered as he leaned close to me.

'They are not all boys,' I said, nodding towards two children reading in the corner. The girls, both wearing rather drab dressing gowns, were on medication and neither had any hair.

Tony made no further comment, just gave a tight, understanding smile. I didn't mention that Lucy's hair was filling her hairbrush every morning, that I feared that she would look just like the other girls very soon.

Yanni was the first to mention Christmas. 'I put the tree up in Rhodes, Mum. Got the new one I had promised Lucy. It's great, she'll love it,' he said, not wanting to look me in the eye.

I choked back the tears.

Don't worry. She'll see it next year.

Monday 31 December

So many days and I haven't written. It's already the last day of 2001. We are at my in-laws.

Lucy was discharged from the hospital on Friday afternoon, 21 December, her first dose of chemotherapy behind her. We were both excited to be getting out of the clinic, for Lucy to be off medication, away from the doctors and nurses, but I did have a nagging feeling without the security the hospital offered.

If Lucy felt something similar she didn't show it. Although tired and weak after the chemo she was dying to spend time with her brothers and to get away from me.

It hasn't been easy. Ten tense days of watching my little girl fight this demon; ten days of seeing her nose, mouth and bottom invaded by herpes, while oozing sores on her lips left her unable to open her mouth. Lucy has been extremely angry and indifferent, uncooperative away from the hospital, refusing to take the medication her doctors have prescribed.

She does take it in the end but it's difficult, a constant battle that leaves me drained and feeling horrible, a tough mother constantly at odds with her sick daughter. I know what I am doing is right but Lucy runs from me as if my touch, my hug, scorches her skin. She bolts straight into someone else's arms and that hurts.

There is, however, no alternative. I watch her face all day and it haunts me all night in my dreams.

Lucy and I were both impatient to leave the hospital, to be away from its routine, to put the treatments behind us for more than two weeks and to return to a home environment. Even a trip to the supermarket with her uncle sounded a treat to Lucy.

We visited Lucy's grandfather and met his wife, who is a small, caring woman who struggles with failing sight and hearing and suffers a tiring, bad limp. She was welcoming, fussed over Lucy and filled her pockets with trinkets, turquoise and small gold beads.

Most days and evenings, however, were spent at home. Even Christmas came and went without much fuss. I was happy to have the boys with us but there was little to celebrate.

There was a special package for me from Sheila, Gro and Sharon. I decided to open it in private. On the top of the package was a bankbook, an account my friends opened on 19 December with a 50,000 drachma (147 Euro) deposit and a note advising me to check with the bank whenever I could.

Sitting on the bed in my nephew's bedroom (poor Manolis, he had been relocated to share with his older brother) I opened the present. There were top-up cards for my mobile phone, packets of peanuts and six miniature bottles of whisky.

'In case of emergency', the card said.

Thank God I was alone because I couldn't stop crying.

⁓

I spent time on my nephew's computer catching up with family and friends and also learning something about Lucy's nasopharyngeal carcinoma.

Dear me, just the words seemed frightening.

Before leaving TAO I'd asked her specialist for the details of her biopsy. Stupid me, I had worried myself sick over requesting the papers but he immediately arranged to have them translated into English so I could try to understand the terms and send them off for further comment.

The report remained daunting even though I found some explanations on the Internet. The official biopsy report on the cervical lymph nodes removed from Lucy's neck detailed: 'One lymph node measuring 0.7 x 0.3 x 0.2 cm. At dissection the cut surface is whitish of soft consistency. Two lymph nodes measuring 2 x 1 x 1 cm and 2.5 x 1.5 x 0.8 cm. At dissection their surface is whitish of hard consistency. Three lymph nodes measuring 0.5, 0.7 and 0.8 cm were separately sent.'

The report continued. 'The histological examination [my first check on the Internet: histology is the study of the microscopic anatomy of cells and tissues of plants and animals. This test provides data to "delineate cause and progress of diseases that impair body function"] showed metastatic deposits [metastasis, or displacement, is from the Greek words μετά = next + στάσις = placement, metastatic disease is the spread of a disease from one organ to another non-adjacent organ] in all six lymph nodes of a nasopharyngeal carcinoma non-keratinizing undifferentiated type (Type III according to WHO). The two lymph nodes measuring 2 and 2.5 cm were fully invaded by the carcinoma. The fibrotic lymph node capsule and the adjacent fibro fatty tissue are also invaded. Vascular invasion of veins and arteries of medium size in the fibro fatty tissue is observed.'

Other details followed. There was also a mention of Epstein Barr. I realised I had a lot to learn. My first search was for nasopharyngeal carcinoma in children. I waited with the feeble hope that nothing would appear but the screen filled with page after page of information on the disease that Lucy was fighting.

I felt pathetic; the other part, however, remained glued to the screen.

I discovered some good, basic information on the American Physician website (www.aafp.org/afp/2001/0501/p1785.html).

————————

Nasopharyngeal carcinoma is a relatively rare form of cancer, known as NPC. It's found in southeast China, some parts of Africa and Asia. Its victims are usually elderly.

What is nasopharyngeal cancer?

Nasopharyngeal (say: nay-zo-fair-in-gee-al) cancer is a tumor that develops in the nasopharynx (say: nay-zo-fair-inks). The nasopharynx is the area where the back part of your nose opens into your upper throat. This is also where tubes from your ears open into your throat.

Who might get nasopharyngeal cancer?

Nasopharyngeal cancer is rare. You are most likely to get

this cancer if you or your ancestors came from southern China, particularly Canton (now called Guangzhou) or Hong Kong.

You are also more likely to get this cancer if you are from a country in Southeast Asia, like Laos, Vietnam, Cambodia or Thailand.

What causes nasopharyngeal cancer?

One possible cause is eating salt-preserved foods (like fish, eggs, leafy vegetables and roots) during early childhood. Another possible cause is the Epstein-Barr virus. This is the same virus that causes infectious mononucleosis, which is called mono. You may also inherit a tendency to get nasopharyngeal cancer.

What are some signs of nasopharyngeal cancer?

If you have nasopharyngeal cancer, you might first notice a lump in your neck. You might have trouble hearing in one ear, or you might have nosebleeds, headaches, ringing in one or both ears, or you might feel a change in sensation over one side of your face. You may have a heavy running nose.

I read that paragraph again and felt the blood drain from my face. I felt faint, strange. Why hadn't the first doctor in Rhodes recognised these signs?

I pictured his face and could have strangled him. I read on.

How can my doctor tell if I have nasopharyngeal cancer?

Your doctor might use endoscopy (say: in-dos-ko-pee) to try to see the cancer. For this exam, a thin tube with a small camera on the end is put into your nose. This lets your doctor get a closer look at the cancer tumor.

Then I understood what the ear, nose and throat specialist was looking for. He had known before surgery that something was drastically wrong.

During endoscopy, your doctor might take a small piece from the tumor (a biopsy sample). The piece of tumor is then sent to a lab where it is looked at under a microscope.

Your doctor might also send you to have MRI (magnetic resonance imaging). This exam is done to see how big the tumor is.

How is nasopharyngeal cancer treated?

Many people with nasopharyngeal cancer can live normal lives. Cure is more likely if the cancer has not spread to other parts of the body … radiation is quite successful in treating cancer in the nasopharynx … the patient might also need to have chemotherapy … radiation and chemotherapy can make you feel tired and sick to your stomach, can cause headaches …

The more I read the worse I felt.

I opened another site for more information on signs of the cancer although there it stressed that 'nasopharyngeal carcinoma causes signs and symptoms that may suggest a variety of diseases and conditions. That fact, combined with the hidden location of the nasopharynx, means most people aren't diagnosed with nasopharyngeal carcinoma until the cancer has spread.'

A site from the Mayo Clinic detailed the biopsy method (see www-cgi.cnn.com/HEALTH/library/DS/00756.html')

Your doctor may also use the endoscope or another instrument to take a small tissue sample (biopsy) to be tested for cancer. Beyond diagnosing nasopharyngeal cancer, a biopsy also tells your doctor the type of nasopharyngeal carcinoma you have. Nasopharyngeal carcinoma is divided into three types based on the appearance of the cells when viewed under a microscope. Your doctor factors in your type of nasopharyngeal carcinoma when selecting your treatment.

Staging
Once the diagnosis is confirmed, your doctor orders other tests to determine the extent (stage) of the cancer, such as:

- **Magnetic resonance imaging (MRI).** MRI helps show whether the cancer has expanded to nearby soft tissues in the head and neck.
- **Computerised tomography (CT).** CT scans show whether the cancer has expanded into the surrounding bone.
- **Bone scan.** A bone scan is used to determine whether cancer has spread (metastasized) to other bones in your body.
- **Chest x-ray or CT scan.** X-ray or CT scan of the chest may show whether cancer has metastasized to the lungs.
- **Lymph node biopsy.** Doctors check the lymph nodes in your neck (cervical nodes) for signs of cancer by performing a biopsy. In some cases you may undergo surgery to remove an entire lymph node through a small incision in the skin. Once your doctor has determined the extent of your cancer, he or she assigns it a stage. The stage is used along with several other factors to determine your treatment plan and your prognosis.

The stages of nasopharyngeal carcinoma include:
- **Stage 0.** The cancer is limited to the lining of the nasopharynx. Also called nasopharyngeal carcinoma in situ.
- **Stage I.** Cancer is confined to the nasopharynx.
- **Stage II.** Cancer may have spread beyond the nasopharynx to the nasal cavity or to the soft tissues of the throat, including the soft palate, the base of the tongue or the tonsils. Or cancer has spread to the lymph nodes on one side of the neck and may or may not have spread to the soft tissues of the throat.
- **Stage III.** Cancer has spread to the lymph nodes on both sides of the neck and may or may not have spread to the soft tissues of the throat. Or cancer has spread to the throat and the lymph nodes on one or both sides of the neck. Or cancer has spread to nearby bones and the lymph nodes on one or both sides of the neck.

———

There was a lot to read, far too much to take in during one sitting, especially after all the days and nights in the clinic. I had been reading for almost two hours, switching pages, checking different sites. Exhausted,

I rubbed my eyes and stopped, marking the sites for an evening in the future. Maybe then I would be calmer, my heart wouldn't be racing and I would be more rational about the fate of that original doctor.

Every three days Lucy had to check at TAO for blood and urine tests and to have the fluid replaced on the Hickman I changed and cleaned every day at home. The first change, away from the guiding hands and eyes of the TAO nurses, had been difficult. Lucy lay on Manolis' bed, glaring at me. She knew that I was shaking, not just my hands, my whole body. She yelled and mocked as I tried to put on the surgical gloves, desperate to keep everything sterile and clean.

'Don't touch me, you're useless!' She spat the words out, looked at me with eyes blazing with hatred and distrust. I was hurt and humiliated but had to push my feelings aside, reminding myself once again how she might be feeling.

The patch was changed every day after her shower, part of the daily routine, and it rarely drew a comment.

I was getting used to her tempers. What I couldn't get used to were her eating habits. She still wasn't touching food. After nearly a week without eating I was frantic and called Lucy's specialist.

'I'm worried. She must be really hungry and yet she's not eating anything.'

'Don't force her to eat,' he said. 'Lucy will eat when she is ready and able to; be patient and don't worry.'

She tried a little soup and crumbled feta cheese. It was pathetic and heart wrenching to watch her nose twitching at the smell of food that she wouldn't or couldn't eat. Lucy had lost weight; she was thin and seemed to be fading away. The solid, strong thighs and calves, testament to hours of pedalling through the moat and the Old Town streets on her racy little mountain bike, had disappeared; a thin neck and gaunt little face all that remained of her cheeky round-faced grin. Her eyes were huge and sad.

Lucy weighed just over 20 kg.

Ointments and antibiotics helped clear the herpes and cold sores but I had no idea what her throat looked like. Her doctor had said that what was visible was just one part of the problem.

My other major problem was Lucy's hair. My initial feeling of panic had changed little, although I tried not to show it as the hair came away in my hands in the shower. It was everywhere, all over her pillow, on her clothing, little trails wherever she sat. I gathered it back in a braid but even that was difficult.

Lucy notices but I don't think she realises that she will lose her hair. I don't know what to say to her. I know I should be talking to her but I can't. I open my mouth and nothing comes out, the simple truth is that I can't stand being the one to tell Lucy that she is going to look like all the other children in TAO. She hates me enough at the moment.
We don't talk about the clinic. I can't.

It's strange the way people cope, or don't cope, with cancer.
For some, just saying the word is impossible. Lucy's aunt doesn't want the boys to know that Lucy has cancer and has told them that she has a strange bug, one that came from somewhere in Africa. I guess that could be partly true according to what I have read online. But the boys aren't stupid. They've seen the other children in the clinic, they sat with Lucy wired up to her drugs and they are seeing the daily changes in her appearance.
We walked together after the hospital visit and I tried to explain the situation, Lucy's illness and the odds of recovery. They know as much as I do now and although many will damn me for telling them, I don't care. They are old enough to know the truth.

A different problem waited when I returned to Anthousa. Yorgos and his family had heard about the bazaar. My in-laws were extremely angry about the love and charity that had been shown, and demanded to know why I had arranged such a thing. They made me feel guilty and awkward, when I should have been enjoying the love and support of my amazing friends. I was too shocked to care or hear what they said. I just wanted Lucy to get better and for us to get back to normal.

Within hours Yorgos had decided to return to Rhodes, supposedly, to set up a new business. I was relieved as he had been drinking early every morning, we weren't getting on at all and I started to feel that his presence wasn't really helping Lucy.

In the midst of all these worries something pretty amazing happened. Rather typically, it started with something I didn't want to do.

My sister-in-law had promised Lucy a trip away from Anthousa, a drive to a monastery dedicated to Saint Ephraim. To be honest I was dreading it and was not at all happy as we all squashed into her car at the start of a 40-minute drive along the coast. Saint Ephraim, known for his healing abilities, was a new name for me on the long list of Greek saints.

I have always been put off by the stifling icon-filled Greek Orthodox churches and was pretty skeptical about the visit to the monastery. What good could it do? Lucy wasn't enthusiastic about going and complained throughout the journey. She had just about had enough when we turned off the main road and my brother-in-law wound our way through thick trees up the hill to the monastery. For a few minutes I felt we were going back in time and I prepared myself for the solitude of a small chapel on the hill. I was not ready for what greeted us: a carpark of vehicles and, lining the monastery entrance, street traders selling small icons, bracelets, crosses and souvenirs. Lucy was tired and didn't have the strength to manage the gravel and the steps so I carried her. What a shock. I couldn't have comfortably picked her up a month ago and today she was as light as a feather. I carried her up the steps and into an open courtyard, which we crossed, and moved to the left, into the church entrance.

I carried Lucy into the church and put her down close to the sarcophagus holding the remains of the saint.

What happened next is a blur.

Tears streamed down my face as the atmosphere of that small chapel overwhelmed me. I tried to pray but nothing came, my prayers remained unformed, without words. I felt totally alone. No, that's wrong. I sensed a presence, an incredibly strong presence, something that was beyond description and possibly beyond my beliefs.

I don't remember Lucy's movements. I heard her talking with her aunt and her brothers but I didn't react. I was strangely calm. Everything was still until someone touched my arm and said we were leaving. I looked for Lucy and saw her walking out of the chapel. She was with her aunt and they stopped to take a tiny corked bottle of blessed oil and to buy small Saint Ephraim medals.

I stood at the entrance and watched Lucy as she walked across the courtyard and, with a little help, down the steps towards the car. She was walking normally, chatting and laughing with the boys.

I didn't speak during the drive home. I didn't want to lose the feeling of hope that was banging its way through my racing heart.

I am writing this and watching the clock. I can hardly wait for midnight and 2001 to end. Not my year and definitely not Lucy's.

2 January 2002

Welcome to 2002 and a New Year. It started with presents and champagne at midnight and a sleepless night wondering what we were pretending to celebrate; the hapless year we had left behind or the year that was just starting.

The first day of the New Year got off to a late start. I was making a coffee when Lucy appeared.

'You just having coffee, Mum?' Lucy was used to my breakfast.

'Yeah. What do you feel like, milk or tea?'

Shaking her head, Lucy screwed up her nose and started opening her aunt's kitchen cupboards. Within seconds she was eating again.

It was a bizarre, extreme situation. One minute she wasn't eating anything and the next she was like a little rabbit, sniffing the food, trying everything, eating all the time, literally shoving pizza and peanuts into her mouth. I thought she would start with yoghurt, soup, something soft, but no, she knew what she wanted and that was anything that she found in front of her!

What a relief. Lucy was ravenous. Cornflakes and fried eggs for a late breakfast followed by a proper meal at midday. She napped in the afternoon but wanted to be woken to eat. If I hadn't been feeding her appetite I would never have believed it.

Lucy's hair is coming out by the handful and there are bald spots that I can't hide or disguise any longer.

At shower time she reminds me of a little bird. Standing under the hot water, her face glowing and happy, she seems to forget about everything. She closes her eyes, turns her face up to the warm, comforting showerhead and just stands there, revelling in the sensation of the water tumbling over her head and body.

I make the most of her closed eyes and gather up the handfuls of hair so she won't see them clogging the plughole.

Getting out of the bath Lucy avoids the mirror, having just a quick look when she is dried and dressed. A shadow passes over her little face, a tight smile.

'I'll be just like Alexandros soon. At least we won't have to worry about nits, eh Mum?'

Her words and her strength break my heart as I kneel down. Our faces are level. Lucy's eyes are full of hurt, a hurt that a seven-year-old child shouldn't have to feel. I wrap her in my arms and for a short moment we are as we used to be. It doesn't last though and Lucy pulls away to slam her way out of the bathroom.

5 January 2002

Saturday morning. We should have been in hospital yesterday but in a rather macabre turn to this story we are snowed in. Snowbound in Athens, something unheard of, something that never happens ... seems I have heard that phrase or something like it many times recently.

Lucy is enjoying it, laughing with her brothers and cousins while I feel strange, confined. I need time on my own and now with this damned snow I can't get out of the back door let alone away from the house. I feel like I'm suffocating and it's driving me mad.

Lucy's hair was awful this morning, matted like a bird's nest. Maria combed it, virtually accusing me of causing the problem. Guess someone has to take the blame. It's obvious that Lucy will lose all of her hair, all those curls that everyone would comment on. I wanted to curse them all. Of course, that feeling passed.

Lucy seems incredibly strong about it all, listening to a lot of ridiculous ideas from her aunty and grandmother. Shit! Often lost for words, I fear my patience is growing thin.

I'll be glad to get into the hospital again.

How stupid does that sound?

It's like fate once again that she hasn't started this second round of treatment.

I want my own world back.

I want Lucy's world back.

I want her back to normal, no matter what it takes.

Sunday 6 January

It's still snowing, heavily, and I am concerned about how we will get to the hospital for Lucy's second chemo treatment. This house is completely snowed in; there has even been an emergency bread and milk delivery by the local authority to ensure that people are not left without food. It's unbelievable. Even the weather is against us now.

The fluid in Lucy's Hickman must be changed but it seems I am the only one worried about it. She's in great form, eating, eating and eating, happy, laughing and confident, not at all bothered by her hair, which is a straggly mess, a few wisps left around her face with a dishevelled, matted plait, a Mohawk mockery of her wonderful blonde hair.

Monday 7 January

Lucy's second treatment started at midday. She was fine, very reluctant to take her hat off this morning, but later joined her friends in the playroom and didn't want me near her.

Getting here was a performance.

While a lot of the snow had been cleared in central Athens, the outskirts remained isolated and Anthousa was no exception. With her second chemotherapy looming and the need to change the fluid in the Hickman, Lucy had to get to hospital. My in-laws' car was snowbound and emergency numbers shown on television were not available in our area. In the end we sought the help of the local authority and their four-wheel drive vehicle. The snow was still more than knee deep outside the house with roads and footpaths indistinguishable under a blanket of virgin snow. Normally it would have been breathtaking, but this morning it was just something else to worry about, an extra burden.

After talking with the local authority drivers we had to carry Lucy from the house, down the hill to the main road, normally a ten-minute walk. Yorgos carried Lucy and I struggled along in their footsteps lugging two bags of clothing and necessities for the hospital. Lucy wanted to walk, to taste the snow, and she was determined to play. Looking at me over her uncle's shoulder she kept up a constant banter.

'Please Mum, let me just play in it for a moment. Please Mum I won't get wet, nothing will happen to me. Mum! Just let me walk in it. That's all I want to do. Mum, don't be so mean. Pleeease!'

I was scared she would slip or fall so I ignored her pleas and we trudged on.

It was quite an effort. My arms were burning from the weight of the bags by the time we reached the waiting jeep that took us to the main road. We quickly hailed a taxi into Central Athens. In heavy jackets, gloves, boots covered in clinging snowflakes, we bundled into a hot, air-conditioned TAO clinic. We looked ridiculous.

A finger-prick blood test and Lucy was admitted once again to TAO, in the big day treatment room because all the other smaller rooms were full. I had a Scottish lady, Eleanor, next to me. Her 14-year-old son, Pandelis, had a brain tumour and was wired to machines I hadn't seen in TAO until then. He didn't look good.

Alexandros and his mum, Joanna, were in the same room. Good news for us at least, as Lucy and I both enjoyed their company.

Lucy's specialist was pleased with her progress. 'Lucy's surprisingly strong and she's determined. That's good,' he said, smiling at my face, which told him I knew too well what her determination could lead to.

'There will be a third chemotherapy after this one and then Lucy will have radiation treatment', he added, before continuing on his morning rounds.

Once settled in TAO I hurried off to buy some things Lucy and I needed. Digging in my bag for my wallet I found the bank book that my friends had sent from Rhodes. I'd heard that my friends' bazaar had been a success but no one had told me the outcome. I had forgotten all about it until then. I turned the small bank book over, ready to throw it back into my bag, when a Commercial Bank sign caught my eye on the opposite street corner. I crossed the road to join a small queue and minutes later handed the book to the teller and requested an update.

I imagine we both expected a quick print out. Our eyes locked as her printer clicked its way through the first page and she had to turn again and again as the printing continued. The teller peered at her computer screen, an incredulous look on her face, as she handed me the bank book.

'Umm, there you go,' she said. 'The total amount is in Euros and drachmas as, I am sure you know, we have already changed currency with the New Year.' She spoke very slowly, almost sounding out the words.

'It's okay. I speak Greek, don't worry, I understand,' I said, groping to find my reading glasses to study the line of deposits. From 147 Euros on the first page I turned to the new total. Three million drachma, 8303 Euros!

I looked at the teller, she looked at me. I couldn't stop the tears streaming down my cheeks. My hands were shaking and I barely moved my head when she asked if I needed anything else. I felt myself smile in thanks and stumbled out of the bank, amazed at what had happened. I stood near the entrance, read and reread the amount. Good God! How had they done that, so much money to help me with Lucy?

I took a deep breath and wiped away the tears. I felt totally overwhelmed and leaned against the bank wall to catch my breath. Thank you. Thank you.

The money would help improve Lucy's life once she was out of hospital and well again. I felt positive, strong, convinced that she would get better. My mind raced. I would find her a new house and be able to provide whatever she needed ...

Tuesday 8 January

It's late evening and we've had a difficult day.

Lucy is on the chemo and has been sick, her confidence quickly shattered with the first bout of vomiting. She's snappy and difficult and has me wishing I had company, someone who could share this with me. Maybe then it would be easier to cope.

The TAO dayroom was busy and full after the arrival of a noisy demanding Albanian boy named Vasilis this morning and, in the early evening, a little girl from Coskinou in Rhodes. She looked very much like Tania, although she could talk. Her mother and aunt, both young and pretty blondes straight from the pages of a fashion magazine, looked stressed but comfortable in the clinic. We talked briefly, long enough for me to understand that this little girl had been through it all before. Her cancer had returned too quickly.

Pandelis woke for a short time. How should I describe what he was going through? He wasn't a child; he was a young man, hidden in a body that his illness had swollen out of all normal proportions. It had changed his looks, invaded his brain, and stripped him of his right to enjoy his teenage years. He communicated with his eyelids, answering his mother's questions by opening and closing his eyes. I watched mother and son together and wondered where Eleanor got her courage from. When Pandelis drifted back to sleep we talked, filling in details of one another's backgrounds. Eleanor told me in a few words that her son's battle was nearing its end. She knew there was little else the doctors could do for him.

'I don't know what to do anymore,' she said. 'It's not fair. Pandelis doesn't deserve this, no child does.' Her eyes filled with tears and we turned away from each other, she to her lifeless son and me to my sleeping daughter, flushed with a slight temperature that was running through her body with the drugs.

And people keep telling me to pray, to believe in God.

What have these little souls done to deserve such treatment? Can someone tell me what they have done?

I am getting used to sharing Lucy's bed and surviving on very little sleep. It's always late when I doze off and early when I wake to shower before the ward really comes to life. I keep thinking about how things have changed. My life, Lucy's life, our everyday routines have changed so drastically and yet ...

I am aware of the hours passing, albeit slowly, but they do pass. The bottles of Lucy's medication empty and are replaced, morning runs into afternoon, evening into night.

Acceptance. There is no alternative.

Wednesday 9 January

Lucy continued with her second treatment, vomiting a few times but nothing like the first round. It didn't seem to set her back so much and she was enjoying the company of the other TAO children, especially during the playroom hours.

Sad and sullen in the morning, turning her nose up at food, her back to me and the nurses, Lucy was unapproachable until she heard the girls' voices. Then she was off her bed in an instant, tugging at the trolley and the swaying bottles, bumping her way across the corridor and laughing with Alexandros, who jostled her at the door.

Within minutes they were busy, little heads bent over their paintings, oblivious to their surroundings. The children paid no attention to their frames and medication, the jangling bottles that clashed together in a tangle of tubes, the computers sounding off if the medicine had run its course. Their illness and problems were forgotten as the girls taunted and tempted them into songs, smiling as the little faces lit up with grins and laughter.

Lucy didn't need me and I spent an hour or so with the parents. Okay, I yo-yoed, in and out of the ward in fear that she might have felt left alone. She didn't of course. It was then that I noticed that Panayiota had been moved into a private room after her mother was told, rather bluntly, that her young daughter was on a one-way road.

'The doctors virtually told me that only a miracle could save Panayiota,' Maria said, drawing heavily on her cigarette as we sat on the TAO steps.

I look at Panayiota and can't bear to think that she is dying. She is fighting, doing everything the doctors tell her, but she is dying, slowly and surely.

In the dayroom we got to know Dimitri. He is a year older than Lucy. His mother is Smaro and she is probably around my age. Dimitri is a quiet little boy, with large, round eyes and, every now and then, the biggest smile. I watched him talking to his mother and was amazed at the love and tenderness, the glow that surrounded them. Smaro was also quiet, sitting on the side of his bed reading, coaxing him to his food. She disappeared every now and then for a cigarette, but was never away for long.

They were close to Alexandros and Joanna. They were, God help them, TAO regulars.

I continued to sit and watch, learning and, occasionally, in conversation, stealing a little of their strength and courage.

———

During the afternoon members of the popular Olympiakos basketball team visited the clinic to spend time with an older boy who, apparently, after months without any problems, had to return to TAO. Maria told me that 17-year-old Antony was very depressed and someone had arranged for the team's visit in the hope of cheering him up.

They arrived armed with extra presents for TAO's other patients and, who knows? They didn't expect to find so many youngsters suffering from cancer? Or they just got their calculations wrong? Whatever, their visit was rather ill-planned as there were not enough gifts to go around and many children were left out. I noticed it straight away with Lucy. She was happy in the playroom and content in her friends' company. However, when the team left she and others were unapproachable, bitter and hurt.

Late in the evening the on-call doctor checked the ward. Sofia Polyxronopoulo was the attractive doctor I'd met the evening before Lucy was moved to TAO. She noticed that Lucy wasn't on good form. 'Hey Lucy, what's wrong? Where's that wonderful smile of yours?'

I explained that Lucy had missed out on the gifts.

'Ah, don't let that worry you Lucy. You have so many gifts of your own you don't need a Barbie doll to make you feel better.' Lucy turned to look at the doctor.

'You've been given the gift of joy. I've watched you, and others have noticed what you can do. You make people smile, they're happy when you are near them, and they want your company. You've also been gifted with courage and a determination that,' she added with a smile, 'probably comes from having to cope with those boisterous older brothers, eh?'

Lucy brightened. She was listening closely to the doctor.

'You know, you and I have a lot in common. We are both islanders, both from the Dodecanese (Twelve Islands). I'm from Calymnos originally. We islanders are born strong, we have to be, so forget about these basketball players and give me that smile that Panayiota has told me so much about.'

Lucy grinned.

'There, that's better ... and while we're talking, Lucy, why don't you do something about your hair. I think I would if I were you! You know us ladies, we all want to look our best ...'

I could have hugged that amazing woman. She succeeded in brightening Lucy and broaching a subject that Lucy would not talk about: her hair. It's awful. It's a straggly rat's tail and is all that remains of her beautiful curls. There are no low mirrors in TAO so Lucy can't see what it looks like. Maybe she doesn't care; maybe she just wants to keep whatever is left.

I don't raise the subject.

But someone else did.

Lucy found a new friend in Tula, the pretty little aunt from Koskinou. Perched on the side of the bed, she sat with Lucy after the doctor had left. They talked about Rhodes, their friends, Lucy's school, and her hair.

Tula said she was a hairdresser (she wasn't) and the two made a pact to cut Lucy's hair. 'The plait,' Tula said, 'has to go.'

Thursday 10 January

I didn't expect Lucy to wake with her hair as her first thought this morning, but she was up early, woke Tula and demanded the promised new look.

'Okay, right ... let me have a coffee first Lucy and we'll do it. I also need to find my scissors ...' she said, widening her eyes slightly as she looked across at me. I got the message. Tula, of course, didn't have any scissors. I borrowed some from one of the nurses, passing them on to Tula without Lucy seeing.

'Okay, Lucy. I'm ready when you are. Where do you think is best for your haircut?'

Lucy shrugged her shoulders and pointed to the pokey dayroom toilet.

'Why not?' Tula said, suppressing a smile. We – Lucy, her frame, Tula and I – tried to fit ourselves comfortably into the lavatory without making too much noise and without too many giggles that could wake the rest of the ward. The harder we tried not to make a sound the noisier we became. Lucy's frame banged on the door and got stuck near the sink. Tula pulled it slightly, lost her balance and sat back on the toilet.

'I'll wait out here,' I suggested, trying desperately not to laugh.

'No! I want you in here Mum. I can't go through this without you.' Lucy was adamant and I squeezed in, just managing to close the door. We couldn't really move so Tula and I had to change places. I sat on the toilet while she took command of the makeshift salon.

'Are you ready Lucy?'

Lucy looked up at Tula and nodded rather solemnly. The plait was attached by a few hairs, nothing more. One quick snip and it was gone. Lucy's early morning haircut took little more than a moment. There were only a few wispy hairs left to frame Lucy's beautiful face.

Full of smiles at first, Lucy lost her confidence when Vasilis commented on her new look. A knitted hat was pulled on low over her forehead and she wore it all day until Alexandros mischievously tugged it off her head this evening.

'Ah, come on Luce, what's the hat for? None of us have got any hair so throw it away. You don't need it in here.'

It was not a good day for Tula's niece. She was very restless following a convulsion during the night, after which her bed was screened off from the rest of the dayroom.

By late evening Lucy was feeling better. The sickness had stopped and she had picked at a packet of baked rolls. She even joined a birthday party on the ward.

Phillip, a quiet little blond boy, remarkably independent and well behaved, another leukemia patient, was two today. His French-born Greek mother, Barbara, was quite a character. She was always talking on her mobile, Greek, English, French, usually in one sentence. She was separated, had another little boy at school and was constantly running between her home and the hospital. She was blonde, bubbly and bright, but I wondered if her boldness was a façade.

Lucy picked at a savoury and sipped at a Sprite at the birthday party, but she didn't sit for long and was on her bed early, possibly feeling the effects of the treatment.

'Are you okay? Do you want anything? Do you want me to read a story? We could draw together if you like?'

'Go away. That's what I want!'

I waited until Lucy was asleep and, after checking her temperature and the dripping medication and ensuring the Hickman lines were clear, finally slid beside her on the bed. I didn't want to wake her and I tried not to move. I was tired but sleep did not come easily.

Friday 11 January

We wake to a sunny day at last. It's always warm in the clinic, sometimes too hot, and quite a shock if I venture outside to the kiosk. This morning it's nice outside, the sunshine and almost a spring feel about the day put me in a good mood, a better frame of mind.

Lucy is good, without the vomiting she's coping well, but she's homesick. She wants to see her father, her brothers and her friends. I'm probably the only person she doesn't want to see!

TAO news is not good. Little Elena's condition is deteriorating and Eleanor's Pandelis faces surgery yet again.

Sunday 13 January

The weekend and thankfully the ward was quiet, probably because noisy Vasilis and his poor aunt were sent home. Phew, what a handful he was. Older than the other children, aggressive and loud, Vasilis wouldn't even get up to go to the toilet, he just settled to wet the bed and he gave his aunty a hard time. Did he do it all on purpose? I couldn't tell. He was angry, with himself, with his family, with everyone it seemed. Who could blame him? From what I could gather he hadn't had much of a life so far, and his illness was just another blow.

Whenever he talked to Lucy I noticed he smiled and his face changed, softened. The darkness and anger faded and, apart from his shiny hairless head, he looked like a healthy, normal 12-year-old boy ready for mischief and adventure. His only adventure in TAO was to haul his trolley out in the sitting room, bullying and tormenting his aunt and the nurses along the way.

He didn't tyrannise Lucy though, his voice was soft and sweet when he talked to her and he gave her a fancy pearl necklace before leaving the ward yesterday.

There is another little Albanian boy, Josef. Routina, his larger than life mother, sings to Lucy and makes her smile with a Christmas song and her silly ways. Her son is stocky, quiet and angry. He glowers over his eyebrows but when he laughs, boy does he laugh, with his heart, with all of his little body.

Not too many of the kids here like Josef, but I don't think he's as bad as they make out. He's scared, extremely angry, and aggressive if he wakes and his mother is not next to his bed, which is more often than not. Perhaps she leaves him a lot ... whatever, it's none of my business, but he shouldn't be ill and sad.

Lucy remained very unhappy, wanted only her father and turned her back on everyone except Papadakis. He gave her good news. 'All going well, Lucy, you will be out of here this time tomorrow,' he said, arranging an appointment with the hospital's dermatologist to check a rash that looks like little stretch marks that Lucy has developed on her hips. He noted that she wasn't eating again but assured me it was nothing to worry about. Reading my thoughts he added, 'I know that's easier said than done but, believe me, Lucy will eat again when she feels able to.'

I visited Eleanor, who was at her son's bedside in the third-floor surgery ward. Pandelis was asleep and looked surprisingly calm. Eleanor looked shattered. She told me she was okay but her eyes said otherwise. She seemed lost and haunted, like someone who was losing a battle.

Artemis and Tula, on the other hand, looked relieved as little Elena had brightened.

Gro called. My friends' bazaar was still causing problems and Gro was being threatened with a court case. My in-laws, she said, wanted to sue her for publicising Lucy's illness. 'But that's ridiculous,' I told her. 'At the end of the day all anyone wants is the best for Lucy.' 'Well, maybe they've forgotten that,' she said.

Sunday 20 January

I've been lax. Almost a week has gone by since we left the hospital after Lucy's second chemo ... maybe I don't need to write every day when she's doing well.

Before leaving Paidon Lucy saw the hospital's dermatologist who prescribed two creams and a bath scrub for the marks on her sides. That same morning she developed an awful rash around the Hickman line and I was advised to leave it without the sticky protective dressing.

Her doctors prescribed no other medication and, ready to leave the hospital early, we waited in vain for Lucy's uncle to appear. An hour later I decided we would take a taxi, but finding a driver who would take us all the way to Anthousa proved much more difficult than I'd imagined. The longer I tried the more impatient and demanding Lucy became. I was just about at the end of my tether when a driver finally agreed to take us.

Lucy first. As with the days following her first treatment, Lucy suffered from a horrible sore mouth and she was unable to eat, sipping occasionally at a chocolate milk drink. She was irritable and angry, even more so when plans for a trip to Rhodes had to be postponed.

That had been mentioned during the final days of her second treatment. Papadakis had even arranged for a week-long Hickman solution but Lucy wasn't eating and she wasn't strong enough to venture too far from the hospital. I opted to stay in Athens.

She didn't take that well. She was bitter and accusing, her words too strong for a seven year-old. As always, her verbal attack left me speechless and wondering if she would ever love me again.

During our few days in Anthousa, Maria and Yorgos promised Lucy a trip to the monastery that didn't eventuate. They also asked me to limit the shower water and the use of the washing machine was restricted. That apart, the days were routine and I just seemed to tick them off. Hickman check, tick; Hickman change, tick; medication after the usual squabble, tick; eating, improving; general feeling …

Maybe it's just me. I'm worried about Lucy, I'm tired and stressed and I don't feel comfortable here anymore. My in-laws have helped enormously but, hey, we all need space. Lucy's treatment here should end midsummer and that's a long time to stay in someone else's home. I'll look into bringing my Fiat to Athens or possibly staying in the hostel, which is near the hospital.

I've heard a lot about the Elpida hostel from others in the clinic. Elpida is the Greek word for hope. The hostel is operated by a charity formed to assist children suffering from cancer. I have heard only good things about the place; it could be just what Lucy and I need.

Monday 21 January

Lucy's three-day check at TAO was good today; good enough to have the doctors support my idea for a few days on Rhodes.

What a feeling! Lucy and I were both beaming with happiness. There was only one problem; there was no evening flight available so I booked for the next morning. Lucy was angry, put out, and all of TAO heard about it.

'I want to go now,' she screamed. 'You're useless. I want my father. Get out of my sight. I don't even want to look at you!'

That hurt but I could do little about her tirade. We returned to my in-laws for the evening, packed a few clothes and waited to leave for Rhodes on the first flight.

Tuesday 29 January

Once again the days have slid by, not unnoticed but with very little time to sit and write. We have been to Rhodes and are now back in TAO, settled strangely enough in the dayroom, in the same bed by the door.

Let's backtrack ...

The Aegean flight to Rhodes was easy. The hostesses fussed over Lucy with sweets and a load of the little giveaway wet wipes, which she hoards. She rewarded them with a big smile, which seemed to fill her tiny face that was made even smaller by the knitted hat she had pulled down to her eyebrows.

That smile remained as she ran through the airport terminal into her father's arms. She looked better and, as I expected, she didn't want anything to do with me. I went home to the Old Town and Lucy moved in with her father and grandmother in her council flat across the other side of the town.

We were apart for the first time since the middle of November.

Yanni, Tony and Sam were full of smiles, hugs and questions. Each answer prompted another query. They wanted to know everything about their sister, her illness and her future; more than anything they demanded to know when we would be back to stay.

'As soon as Lucy is well again.'

'When will that be, Mum?'

'I'm not sure ... when the treatments are over. Maybe in a few months' time ...'

'A few months! But that's ages.'

Their disappointment made me want to cry. 'Ah, come on. It won't be long and Lucy and I will be back here and you'll be wishing we weren't again.' My attempt to lighten the situation was as feeble as their smiles.

My poor boys. They're fighting their own battle as well.

I spent many hours with them and together we had the little house looking like home, well almost, again.

The paperwork I tackled was not so straightforward. Nothing is ever easy in the Greek bureaucracy's world of rubber stamps and signatures.

I was on the verge of collapse but that didn't matter, as Lucy was smiling, happy to be away from the clinic and to have time with her family and some friends. I saw her every morning to change the Hickman dressing. She was always delighted to see the back of me and spent every night with her father.

On the third day on Rhodes Lucy seemed troubled by phlegm, she was unsettled and her mouth started to look sore again. She wouldn't use the mouthwash prescribed by her TAO doctors and took her other Zovirax medication only after arguments. I didn't want her to get any worse so in a way I was glad our stay on Rhodes was short.

Yorgos and I had just about managed civil conversations over the three days. As long as we were talking about Lucy we were fine, or so I thought, until the last moments of the trip when he was driving us to the airport to return to Athens. He'd offered the ride and I'd accepted, thinking we could talk with Lucy. It would, I thought, be a positive way of leaving Rhodes and heading back to Athens and her third treatment.

But I was wrong. I didn't realise until a few minutes into the journey that he had been drinking. He wasn't drunk but had obviously had just enough to get started. He was driving, we were talking and suddenly, he turned on me.

Hurt, I choked back a response and leaned over to cuddle Lucy, who quickly moved as far away from me as possible. We reached the airport in a strained silence and, of course, Lucy didn't want to leave. She was unhappy and remained poker-faced and unapproachable throughout the flight. She was very tired.

During the flight, I tried to shrug the ill feelings away but no matter what, Yorgos' outburst hurt. I feel awful, angry and bruised. Doesn't he ever wonder how I would manage without my friends?

Lucy's uncle picked us up at the airport. Thank goodness it was late and he and my sister-in-law understood that Lucy and I were worn out. We settled to sleep on a pulled-out divan in Lucy's godfather's small apartment. Lucy was quiet, withdrawn, curled in towards me. We both fell asleep rolling into the middle of the dumpy couch. I woke to Lucy's sobs.

'Mum … Mum, what have I done?' Lucy was kneeling in the middle of the couch and her nightgown was wet.

'Mum, I've wet the bed,' she sobbed.

'Never mind. It's nothing. Don't worry.'

Oh my poor little girl! I wondered what went through her mind and governed her dreams at night. Could a seven year-old with cancer have dreams, or were they all nightmares?

Before starting her treatment today Lucy had an ultrasound on her neck, full urine and blood tests and a triplex heart ultrasound, to check a problem on the Hickman line, which for some reason was blocking, making routine blood tests complicated and time consuming.

Sunday 3 February

Almost a week in TAO and Lucy was nearing the end of her third treatment. She'd suffered some vomiting but, like everything else – moving in to the clinic, the paperwork, getting wired up to the drugs, finding a good trolley frame that ran easily and didn't feel like a faulty supermarket trolley – she was used to it. It was, unfortunately, routine.

Artemis, Tula and Elena were in a private room. Elena had changed, she looked heavier, rarely smiled and communication was limited. Panayiota had also changed, quite dramatically, during our few days' absence. She had lost most of her hair, looked bloated and ungainly and her movements were slower. We sat outside the playroom and she talked to me about Lucy.

'I was sure there was nothing wrong with her when I first saw her. She was so full of life, so beautiful, too special to be sick. I cried when I saw she had lost her curls and looked like all the other kids in here. It's not fair is it?' she said as tears rolled down her cheeks. She wiped them away and looked at me with hurting eyes.

'You know what, Colleen? I believe Lucy is going to be one of the lucky ones. She'll be fine.'

There was a newcomer to TAO, a beautiful little blonde tot from Crete who attached herself to Lucy on her first day in the clinic. Magda arrived in TAO with her mother during a party in the waiting room. All the children were there, squeezed in to form a semi-circle around a clown, who kept them entertained for an hour or so.

Magda was holding her mother's hand as they came through the main door into the TAO lounge. She was quick to drop it when she saw the clown and jumped in to join the party. Literally. One moment she was hanging off her mother's hand and the next she was next to Lucy. Her first impression of TAO was, 'Wow! A party! A clown!' She wanted to be part of it all and didn't even glance at her mother as she squeezed herself in beside Lucy.

'Hi, what's going on here?' she said, bright-eyed and full of surprise. She looked around at the children and concentrated on the clown. 'Wow.'

Magda was quickly part of the 'gang', even though her blonde curls clashed with the shiny bald heads of her new friends. She was confident and somehow happy to be in TAO, though her mother was not. A big, tall woman, she looked wild and unapproachable, larger than life. Somehow I knew this wasn't the case. Magda's mother was scared, very scared, and she looked shattered.

Yorgia was from Crete. We chatted in the corridor and moved to the smoking terrace. She told me that her little girl had a tumour on her kidney. Magda, she said, would not undergo an operation; she was in TAO to begin chemotherapy. Like me, Yorgia had little warning of her daughter's illness.

Heavens, no wonder this poor woman was distraught; she was still bleeding from giving birth to her third child, a little boy, when she learned that she would have to leave him and her older daughter to take her little girl to Athens to see specialists.

Leaving Yorgia I bumped into Artemis. She was pale and had been crying.

'What's up? How's Elena?'

'It's not Elena', she said sobbing. 'It's Pandelis. He died this morning; he never recovered from the surgery. Oh God, poor Eleanor.'

Death seemed to stalk me that day. Later in the evening I heard that a local store owner on Rhodes (I had interviewed him the previous year while researching an article I wrote for a London-based magazine that Martin edited) had lost his 20-year-old son in a freak accident in Athens. Two young men were walking along the footpath en route to a concert when a car sped out of control, mounted the pavement and hit them. One died instantly and the other was in intensive care.

I hardly knew the father and didn't know the boys but I was shocked and shaken by the fatality.

Death is around us all the time at the moment. We seem to be clothed in it, stifled by it. Hearing of this sudden death is so different to the threat we are dealing with all day, every day.

I wonder which is worse, if there is a worse.

Can you ever prepare yourself for death?

Is it better to know and understand that it's lurking rather than suddenly lose your child? I have to stop thinking like this. I can't sleep and during the day I can hardly concentrate.

I've talked with Papadakis about Lucy's next treatment involving heavy radiotherapy. It's not available at the children's hospital. He recommended a specialist at the nearby Saint Savas hospital and arranged a meeting. Leaving Lucy with her friends in TAO, I went alone, following her doctor's instructions.

The Agios Savas Hospital was easy to find and I had no trouble finding Dr Zampaties, who welcomed me into his office. Tall and gangly, with wild curly hair and bulging eyes, he was a bit off-putting at first glance, but his smile was kind and his manner quiet. He read the notes I had carried from TAO and sighed.

'Your daughter is very young. We usually deal with older patients. Phew, I'm not used to dealing with children.' Running his fingers through his thick hair, he turned the pages of Lucy's file, returned to the initial note from the biopsy and sighed again.

'Let me think about the best way to deal with your little Lucy. I'll talk to my colleagues and call you within the next ten days. Then we'll need to meet Lucy and measure her for a mask for the radiation treatment.'

'How long will the treatment last?' I asked as he guided me to the door.

'Six to seven weeks.'

There I was talking about another treatment, six or seven weeks of it, as if it was something totally normal. I really had no idea what lay ahead for Lucy.

Walking back to the clinic I decided to apply for a room at the Elpida hostel. When Lucy started daily radiotherapy I felt pretty sure it would be better for us to be close to the hospital.

Panayiota had stayed at Elpida with her mother. Maria gave me the phone number and I arranged to meet with the head social worker, Dimitri, the next day.

One of the first things Dimitri said to me was: 'Children who stay here get to enjoy Elpida, and believe it or not some don't want to leave.' We took a small lift up to the third floor, where he showed me a typical Elpida bedroom. It was like a twin-bed hotel room, a bit stark, but Dimitri stressed that the kids and mothers tend to make the place their temporary home.

'You and Lucy can decorate your room as you like, as long as there is no structural damage,' he added with a grin. Dimitri explained what papers I needed from the hospital and shook my hand. 'I can't wait to meet Lucy,' he said.

I wandered back from the hostel feeling a lot happier and somehow more positive.

I wondered if Lucy would look forward to meeting him though.

She was spitfire angry on my return to TAO, screaming that I had left her for too long, throwing her prized mobile phone, a gift from her father, in my face as I bent to kiss her. 'I want my father. I don't want to be here with you. I can't stand you!'

It definitely was not the right time to introduce the hostel plan. I felt awful. My mobile buzzed and it was my sister-in-law's turn to have a go at me for something that was said during our few days on Rhodes.

I heard her voice. '… all of Rhodes is talking … gossip …'

'Enough!' For once I opened my mouth. I realised later that what I said to her shocked a few of my new friends at TAO who later admitted that they had never heard me talking like that.

Good for you, they said. You mustn't keep things bottled up. It's not good for you.

It may not be good for me but, as I thought, my in-laws didn't visit for a few days. My only break was a quick dash to the kiosk or the shops and I showered early and quickly, like a thief, in the communal showers down the corridor. I even resorted to washing my undies and Lucy's nightwear in the sink here and drying them over the heater. Not the best but at least our clothes are clean.

We had a visitor from Rhodes. Ingrid was Gro's friend. President of the International Club on Rhodes, she had translated a series of guidebooks I'd written into Swedish. Ingrid was also a cancer survivor.

Ingrid sat on the side of Lucy's bed. 'Do you know how many people on Rhodes are asking after you, Lucy? No? Well, it's pretty amazing. There are a lot of people on the island who love you and your mother very much.

'Even my elderly neighbour wanted to give you a little surprise, something to cheer you up. He gave me this,' she said, handing Lucy a pretty wallet, 'and he insisted that the money inside would be spent on something you really, really want.'

Lucy smiled and put the wallet under her pillow. 'Thanks. I don't really want anything at the moment but I'm sure I'll find something … Hey, Mum, maybe we can buy that GameBoy, eh?'

For a few seconds Lucy had her old look, a cheeky, pretty little girl who had a habit of getting her own way.

'This clinic is nothing like I'd imagined,' Ingrid said. 'There is so much light in here and look at these children. They are all on medication but they're talking and smiling … it's amazing, the atmosphere here is incredible.'

I introduced her to Lucy's specialist, who sat on the bed and chatted with Lucy. 'And that's something special as well,' Ingrid said. 'Look at the way those two interact. I'm impressed!'

I felt it was good for someone else to see what I admired so much in TAO. Ingrid said the International Club was determined to help me financially and that she would arrange the payment of some of the boys' extra lessons on Rhodes.

'That money has been set aside to help you,' she said. 'But you must know that there are some women very much against you on Rhodes. I have no idea where their thoughts come from but they seem to think you and Lucy are having a great time in Athens. I've heard you're living it up, going out to bouzouki, having some kind of holiday and getting other people to pay for it.'

I felt sick. I was livid and, as she talked, my feelings showed.

—

Xenia called into TAO the same evening, armed with a beautiful basket of cookies for me and chocolates for Lucy. 'What are we celebrating?' Lucy asked her. 'Oh nothing, Lucy. I just love that shop. I walk past it every day and often stop to buy something ... as you can see. It's amazing how good chocolate can make you feel,' she chuckled.

I told Xenia about my plans to move into the hostel.

'The problem is that I haven't told Lucy yet.'

'Why is that a problem? She'll love it there.' Lucy returned to sit on her bed.

'Hey Lucy. Your mum was just telling me about Elpida. It will be great if you can stay there. It's like a little hotel and they do loads of things for the kids, trips away, theatre, you'll make even more friends.'

'Sounds great, eh, Mum? When are we moving in?'

Lucy was in a surprisingly good mood after Xenia's visit and I wondered if the chocolate power had worked on her as well.

It's late and I can't sleep. Ingrid's comments keep running through my head. Why on earth would people say Lucy and I were on holiday? I wish we were.

10

Friday 15 February

Many days have passed and I haven't even looked at this diary. I don't know why, sometimes I just don't feel like putting pen to paper, although I know it is also a kind of therapy for me.

Lucy has been in and out of hospital, we've been back to Rhodes and are now settled in the Elpida hostel, biding our time towards an early start tomorrow and another trip to Rhodes to celebrate Lucy's eighth birthday.

Sounds just like that holiday Lucy and I are meant to be enjoying. If you miss out the cancer, the treatments and the hospital.

Lucy finished her third chemotherapy on the evening of Monday 4 February. We left the hospital the following afternoon and flew home for five days.

Once again I hardly saw Lucy as she opted to stay with her dad and her grandmother. In hindsight it was a mistake. Although I was there every day to change the Hickman dressing, I wasn't on hand to check that she was taking enough fluids and to ensure that she was taking good care of her mouth after the powerful chemo.

Lucy knew what she had to do but wasn't careful and the results were ugly, raw mouth sores and a fiery temper.

This time, however, she wasn't just angry; she wasn't well at the same time. She was drinking only milk, had a lot of saliva and phlegm and was vomiting. She was very anti-me, extraordinarily aggressive, and unhappy whenever I was around.

I spent most of my time at the national IKA medical insurance offices and changing my unemployment benefit so I could claim it in Athens. I met with social welfare workers to finalise the cancer benefit payments and generally ran about like an idiot.

⸺

By the time we left Rhodes, Lucy had deteriorated. Her mouth was invaded by sores, and she was down and depressed, not at all interested in food and hardly drinking anything. The flight was a late one so we spent the night with my in-laws. I told them of my plans to move into the hostel and that Lucy had to be in TAO for early blood tests and a magnetic scan.

In the morning I packed a large bag to move into Elpida and Maria, with a night to dwell on our move into the city, was hostile and very defensive.

In the short time it took to go downstairs to get our bag Lucy was in tears.

'I don't think I want to go, Mum. My aunty will look after us here,' she said as her aunt put a protective arm around her shoulders. I took a deep breath; I didn't want to start an argument so I ignored both of them.

That sounds awful, but I did.

I knew what had to be done so I picked up the bags and headed towards the car. Lucy followed and Maria reluctantly agreed to take us to the main road to find a taxi. She definitely was not happy with me.

In the end she had to drive us right to the hostel as the taxis were on strike. Conversation was minimal. Maria remained angry and I felt awkward and somehow at fault in my attempt to make our time in Athens more comfortable – for Lucy and for them. Lucy and I struggled into the hostel and were shown to a room on the fifth floor. I opened the door and Lucy went in.

She was not impressed, not at all.

'Looks just like the hospital here', she said, pulling at the white bedcover, opening and slamming shut the wardrobe and cupboard doors. I dropped the bag in the middle of the big, airy room and we headed straight to TAO for tests.

Lucy was angry and miserable, and her attitude was understandably worsened by the incredibly late 6pm scan. When it was finally over, an exhausted Lucy and I returned to the clinic, ready to head to the hostel, only to hear from the doctor on call that Lucy had to stay in the hospital as her urine tests had revealed a lack of nitrates. Panayiotou was another approachable, handsome man who was, I had heard, a leukemia survivor. However, for Lucy, it was the last straw.

She was beside herself, sad and disheartened as we moved back into the day treatment room, to the same bed as before, as if it had been waiting for us.

Lucy's specialist remarked, 'I'm not getting my usual response from Lucy. The treatments have knocked her, shocked her system and this problem now is like the breaking point. It's understandable that she's so low. I think she needs a break. Lucy needs a treat,' he said, 'a wish … that's it!'

He gave me the phone number for the Make A Wish Foundation in Athens and suggested I call them. I did and two of their volunteers, Mari and Maro, visited Lucy the next evening.

After speaking with Lucy, Maro said, 'Well, Colleen. I explained to Lucy that she could think of three wishes and she was surprisingly quick. She wants to go home. I told her again to think of three wishes and again she was quick. A doll's house, a GameBoy computer game or a painting and drawing kit. Then she changed her mind again. She told me she didn't want anything. She just wanted to go home and that, I'm afraid, is the one wish we can't grant at the moment. I think it's better that we leave Lucy's wish for a while. We can come back when she's feeling stronger, when she's had a chance to think of a wish that really could come true.'

The next afternoon there was another visitor to TAO. Greek pop idol Saki Rouvas visited the clinic to spend time with little Elena, who continued, against all odds, to surprise all the specialists with her will to live.

I've become very close to Artemis and Tula, and the girls have a lot of time for Lucy, who assures them she will play with Elena when she can have visitors again. I think even Lucy knows that's unlikely.

That's just part of the bizarre game that is played here. Every day I ask how Elena is and the sisters smile and shrug. What else can you say? Any changes? Anything new? Any miracle on its way?

Artemis told me that her daughter had fallen for the young star during a visit to Elpida. 'It was amazing to see them together. Elena sparkled when Saki spoke to her and she was lost and lonely when he had to leave. One of the girls at Elpida came up with the idea of contacting Saki in the hope that he might just spark that flame again ...'

The other children, apart from Lucy, waited for Saki at Elena's door, clambering for an autograph or a smile from this strikingly good-looking young man. He was ready to leave when Artemis told him there was another little girl from Rhodes on the ward. He quickly moved into the dayroom and sat on Lucy's bed. 'Hi there Lucy. How come you didn't join the other kids in the corridor? Aren't you feeling well? I've been told you are really pretty and all the boys on the ward are after you. How can I tell if they are right or not if I can't see you?'

Lucy finally gave in and talked with this friendly young star, whose chat and warmth with the children was as genuine as his smile. He is a star on and off the stage.

—————

Yorgia was told today that little Magda could undergo an operation to remove the tumour. It was good positive news. Yorgia brightened and her daughter continued to delight the ward with her antics. We also had good news; an all clear to leave TAO tomorrow. I did, however, have to run like an idiot to IKA doctors in a totally separate hospital to get a prescription for a booster injection that Lucy will be taking for the first time. My health insurance covers all the medical costs while Lucy is in hospital but any medication proposed by her doctors for use out of the clinic must be prescribed by an IKA doctor.

As soon as we had clearance from Lucy's doctors I tried to book a flight to Rhodes. The first available was early Saturday morning so Lucy and I spent our first night together at the hostel.

When we had left our bags at Elpida at the beginning of the week the room seemed rather cold and stark. I had brightened it up with colourful sheets from a local supermarket. With Lucy in the dayroom all week, I was able to run to the hostel each day to take a long shower. I felt slightly more 'me', clean and more independent, even if I was a bit like a thief, in and out, scarcely seeing anyone except the friendly men on the reception desk.

I did meet our 'neighbours'. Antony and his parents were on the same floor, two doors away from our room, so Lucy would have his company at least, and there was a very small baby across the corridor. The other rooms were still and quiet behind closed doors.

Our first sleep at Elpida and, so far so good. Lucy seems quite happy, snug and warm in bed in a big, bright, clean and comfortable room. At the moment she is watching something on television and seems content to be able to work the remote control for both that and the air conditioning.
I feel positive, almost relaxed. I am sure we will be a lot happier here. Life will be easier somehow.

Monday 25 February

We flew to Rhodes extremely early on 16 February. I had worried unnecessarily about getting a taxi from the hostel in the middle of the night; it was all taken care of by Christos, the receptionist here who, like the rest of the Elpida staff, could not have been more helpful.

The following day, 17 February, was Lucy's eighth birthday. Put off by the cold, damp Rhodes weather and my chilly old home, and worried how Lucy would feel seeing her friends and their reactions to the frail little girl who had replaced their robust playmate, I had planned a quiet party. A stream of smiling friends quickly put paid to that idea.

Lucy blew out her candles wearing a heavy jacket and her knitted hat.

She didn't care about the cold, she wasn't concerned with the possibility of germs and infections, she was intent on enjoying her friends' company. What harm could they do? She was crying out for their love and support and they were all willing to give her exactly what

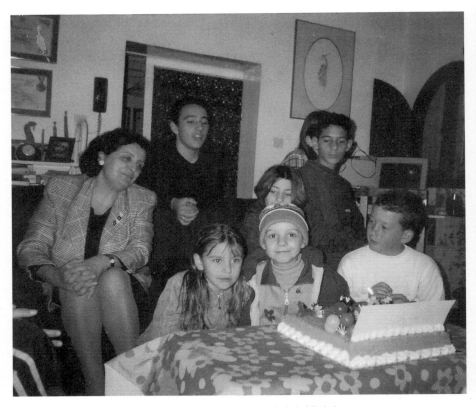

On Rhodes to celebrate Lucy's eighth birthday on
17 February 2002, at the end of her chemotherapy

she needed. Smiles, laughter, hugs. It was obvious that Lucy is a much-
loved, much-missed little girl.

Leaving Rhodes after those busy days wasn't so difficult. There were
no major traumas, although Lucy was badly constipated the last few
days, which really seemed to scare her. We were both relieved when she
finally went to the toilet.

Sheila lent me her laptop so hopefully I'll be able to get online at the
hostel and keep up with everyone instead of running off to the horrible
Internet café opposite the hospital.

We returned to Athens and, for once, I felt ready to help Lucy face
her next hurdle.

Tuesday 26 February

Back at the hostel after an evening at my in-laws. I was dreading it (who knows, they probably had the same feeling) but it was okay. I am indebted for what they have done to help Lucy and me. At the same time I am thankful that we have found our own niche here in Elpida.

Lucy is getting to know the other children here and has a big smile on her face. She has company and is now happily in the lounge, watching a video with Dimitri, who has also moved in to Elpida.

We have a big day tomorrow. It's the first meeting at Saint Savas hospital for Lucy's radiation treatment. I don't know what to expect and fortunately Lucy hasn't asked too many questions.

I often sit and watch her and wonder what's going on in her head. Does she understand her illness? I'm sure she knows more than I do.

Generally she's in very good form, eating normally and full of life, singing, loving, attentive, a little bit difficult only when we shop, as she expects to buy something every time we go out. That's one habit I'll have to break.

She's full of energy and although she lapses into her, 'I want to go to Rhodes, I wish I was in Rhodes,' mode, I'm pretty sure that is completely normal.

Wednesday 27 February

I have just closed my mobile phone after talking to my London friend, Chris, who is planning a trip to Athens. She wants to see us and suggested a long weekend, just the three of us, Chris, me and Lucy, staying in a hotel in central Athens. Sounds a great idea but I have my doubts following a particularly nasty row with Lucy that has rocked my confidence and left me feeling incredibly lonely and lost once again.

The day started well, with an early meeting with Dr Zampaties at Saint Savas. I really wasn't sure where to go and paused in front of the entrance into the main building. I guess we stood out in the courtyard, as people kept turning to look briefly at Lucy, then at me, with long, accusing glares. One woman even hissed at me as she brushed my arm. 'What are you thinking? You're crazy bringing a little girl in here.'

Fortunately Lucy didn't hear her and moments later Zampaties spotted us, introduced himself to Lucy and told us to wait at the coffee shop. I asked Lucy for her impression.

'A bit mad looking ... not angry mad, Mum, weird mad. Did you see his eyes? Do you think there's something wrong with him? If there is something wrong with his eyes how will he see whatever is wrong with me? And his hair Mum. Did you see his hair?'

Dr Zampaties was a new style of doctor for Lucy, who had become used to the more conservative types in TAO. She was right, he did have a kind of mad professor air, but Papadakis had recommended him and that really was enough for me.

A little later, another shorter, English-looking man joined the doctor outside the coffee shop at our meeting. He was commenting on Lucy's type of cancer and said in English, 'Heavens, that's very strange,' looking at Lucy as if she was a ghost. He realised I understood his English and looked extremely uncomfortable.

And I felt sick.

'Why is it so strange? Why are you so shocked by Lucy?' I demanded.

Thanos hurriedly introduced himself and went on to explain that he had only ever seen Lucy's type of cancer in elderly patients. 'I'm sorry. I'm really not used to dealing with children.' He was struggling but his concerned smile was genuine, sincere. He said he was a physicist and would also be working with Lucy.

The men guided us through the hospital corridors, a colourless grey and green maze that I imagined we would have to get used to. Lucy wasn't at all keen on her new surroundings; we were both used to the security of the TAO clinic and being close to children and nursing staff who we knew and for whom we had come to care. This was something totally different. A hospital for adults with cancer and, God only knows, there seemed to be a lot of patients wandering about.

We were shown into a large room, a bit like an operating theatre, with one bed in the middle. Lucy was asked to sit on the bed and I was offered a chair. Zampaties pulled up another chair, close to Lucy. They were face to face as he began talking.

'Lucy, what we are going to do is use this white mesh to make you a mask.'

'What for?' Lucy asked.

'This mask will protect your precious little face during your treatments. It will also keep you from moving your head.'

'Why?'

'Because I'll need you to keep very very still when you start coming here every day. It's hard to describe now, but you'll get used to it. And we'll help you all the time. Now, what I need you to do is lie down here, just lean back and put your feet up. Wow, great trainers Lucy. Where did you get them from?'

Lucy looked down at the shiny pink trainers her best friend had given her for her birthday. 'They're from Rhodes. Georgia gave me them.' Her voice trembled.

'They're amazing', added one of the doctor's assistants, a young dark-haired woman who guided Lucy back on the bed. 'Just lay back and stay as still as you can.'

I was so tense I imagined they could all hear my heart thumping as I watched Lucy, wide-eyed, frightened and anxious – at first. With a little coaxing from Zampaties and smiles from his pretty assistants, Lucy did exactly as she was told as their fast hands patted and stretched the white netting into shape over her face. They won her confidence and Lucy won their admiration and support. Within minutes they had produced a Casper-like mask of Lucy's tiny face.

'Okay, that wasn't so bad,' she declared as the doctors hugged her and helped her off the bed.

'That's enough for today,' Zampaties said. 'I don't want to scare Lucy so we'll just takes things slowly. The mask is important and it's vital that she is not scared of it.' He added that he had scheduled a CT scan at Agios Savas on Friday.

That meant finalising paperwork to cover the cost of the treatment and the scan. Back on my high horse … why, oh why, couldn't this paperwork be easier?

I suggested taking Lucy back to the hostel but no, Zampaties said the national insurance doctors would want to see Lucy to verify the treatment, so a wild goose chase began. First to find the right office in the hospital to stamp the paper from Zampaties (I managed that on the fourth attempt), then off down the busy main road to find an IKA national insurance centre, only to be directed to their main office in central Athens.

It wasn't easy. Lucy was tired and irritable; her co-operative attitude left well behind with the Agios Savas nursing staff. She complained bitterly as I tried to find a taxi, always passing except when you needed one, and promptly told the driver what a useless mother she had.

She didn't understand that I hated all this unnecessary running about more than she did.

At IKA we were blessed with good fortune. The office lady was extremely helpful and sent us immediately to an in-house pediatrician who was tiny, only about as tall as Lucy. She was another godsend as Lucy liked the idea of being examined by someone her own height. She grinned as she was checked by the young, very pleasant doctor, standing on a platform in the grottiest of surgeries with the most amazing view of the Acropolis.

It was somehow bizarre but we were given the necessary paper and laughed together in the taxi back to Elpida.

She is so unsure of me at times. She knows I can do whatever is asked of me and it annoys the hell out of me that she thinks everyone else can do it except me. Guess I should be used to it by now.

Thursday 7 March

So many days and such a lot has happened one way or another.

Lucy has yet to start the radiotherapy but everything is ready for Monday morning. At the moment she is playing with her dolls' house and Barbie dolls and listening to music. Our hostel room is bright with toys and decorations and she is quite happy – for now.

I have to relish these moments because when she is angry Lucy can be really vile. Her alternative to cursing is, 'I am going to call Dad.' It's like saying; 'I am going to report you to the police.' She knows it annoys the hell out of me and I can do nothing to stop that feeling. I get down and lonely.

When I am desperate for a cuddle Lucy is the only one around. She is more likely to bite me than cuddle me.

We have made close friends with Smaro and Dimitri. We usually eat together and have been out shopping and wandering in downtown Athens. Smaro is my age, works in a bank, is serious but funny at the same time. Dimitri has been fighting leukemia and has been sick on and off for three years. There is something – his eyes, his smile, his kindness – very special about him.

Lucy's scan at Agios Savas a week ago was unfortunately much like many of her tests. It took too long and the longer we sat in the waiting area, the more annoyed and anxious Lucy became. When she was finally called into the scan area and asked to lie down to have her Casper mask fitted, she baulked and blankly refused.

I sympathised with Lucy but at the same time felt for the doctors and nurses who really didn't know how to cope with my eight year-old.

'Oh, come on Lucy. Help us a bit on this. We know it's not nice but it's something we have to get right,' Thanos explained.

Helping Lucy to lie back, he and one of the assistants placed the mask over Lucy's face. She struggled and pushed her way to sit upright again.

'No! I can't do that. It's too tight. I can't breathe. Mum!' I moved to hold her hand and the technicians tried again.

Zampaties' turn. 'One more attempt Lucy. Just give us one more and we'll get it right. I promise.' She lay down again and was quiet until I was asked to wait outside.

'No! Mum!' I could see her hand reaching out from the bed.

'Mum!'

'It's okay Lucy, your mother can stay,' said one of the assistants, handing me a heavy protective apron.

I struggled in that room. Lying on the enormous slab-bed, Lucy looked like a little dot under the machine. She did exactly as she was told and didn't move a muscle. I felt so proud and so very, very sad.

Over the weekend we were busy, starting with an outing with Xenia. She picked us up from the hostel in her small car and whisked us off towards Kiffisia, one of the most expensive northern suburbs of Athens.

At Kiffisia we parked with difficulty and then wandered what is regarded by many as the top shopping centre in Greece. An accessory shop was the first stop. Xenia bought Lucy a mauve cap. Lucy was enjoying the shop so Xenia and I moved towards the door, chatting. I told her that Yanni was in Athens on a school trip.

'He's staying in The President, quite close to the hostel, but I haven't seen him yet,' I told her. 'Today they're on an excursion out of Athens, but hopefully we'll get to see him at some stage.'

Leaving the shop we made our way along the main street. Lucy was quick to spot the McDonald's sign.

'Pleeease Mum, can we eat here?'

'No, Lucy there are so many other places.' She pulled a face and I didn't want a scene with Xenia.

'Okay, just a small portion of chips and then we don't have to sit down.'

I joined the queue at the counter, absently reading the back of a group of teenagers' t-shirts. 'Second Senior High School, Rhodes.'

'Hey Lucy, there are kids from Rhodes here', I said, turning to speak to her. I looked straight into Yanni's eyes.

'Mum! What are you doing here?'

'What are you doing here? You're meant to be out of Athens today.'

'The trip was cancelled at the last minute and they brought us here instead. Great timing,' he added, 'now you can pay for my meal!'

That was typical Yanni, I explained to Xenia later when we laughed at the odds of bumping into him in this huge city. Lucy wasn't impressed. In what was becoming a usual mood shift she became very angry and was incredibly rude to poor Xenia, who was only trying to give us a few hours away from our normal routine.

Back at the hostel I was in the dining room, talking to the twins on the phone. 'Say hello to everyone on Rhodes,' I told them as I stood up and moved towards the lift. A striking, thin girl at the next table touched my arm.

'Are you also from Rhodes?' Her question marked the start of a new friendship. Effy, a pretty blonde in her late twenties, introduced herself, her mother and her little boy, Yorgos. A thin, pale child, Yorgos was beginning treatment after an operation to remove one of his kidneys, which had been invaded by a tumour. They were also on the fifth floor, just a couple of doors from our room.

On Sunday morning we had something special to do, somewhere special to go. We had been invited to Magda's christening in the small chapel in the Saint Sofia grounds. Lucy was determined to look her best. She was in good form, happy in new clothes, which were a gift from her godmother on Rhodes, and the matching Kiffisia cap. Little Magda was delighted to see her.

We hadn't seen Magda for a while as Lucy's tests were at Saint Savas and Magda was never about whenever we went into TAO. I had heard about an operation and that Magda had started therapy, but nothing prepared me for the shock when we walked into the church.

Our little blonde angel from Crete, all eyes and a huge grin, was even tinier than before. She had lost her wonderful curls and was completely bald. I fought back tears as I looked at this younger, smaller version of Lucy. I ached to hold her and hug her, but I didn't. I matched her smile and struggled not to show that my heart was breaking.

You don't show the shock.
You just smile.

I told her she was gorgeous, which she was. The christening was wonderful, incredibly sad and touching, and I couldn't hide my tears as this little bundle, with her huge scar from her operation and her covered Hickman, was christened.

Yorgia looked great, totally different from the distant, crushed woman who struggled to get her daughter through the clinic doors a few weeks ago. She beamed confidence, was happy and smiling, crushing me in her arms at the end of the christening. She talked about both our girls being brides.

'We'll see that one day, won't we?' Yorgia asked and looked into my eyes, into my soul. 'We'll laugh at their weddings, think of these and other moments and only we'll know what we are smiling about.'

I spoke with Artemis and Tula and Antony and his mother. Pagona was pale, a shadow of her usual positive self. She quickly told me that Tony would be returning to the bone marrow transplant unit. I tried to cheer her up, but what could I say? Lost for the right words I could only hug her, hoping she could feel my concern.

Lucy's specialist was there, along with lots of other familiar faces, all present for this special hour, one where the clock stopped and usually sad and worried faces smiled for a little warrior.

Lucy wanted to see her aunt so from the hospital we caught a bus to my in-laws where a happy, bubbly Lucy broke the initially strained atmosphere. I hoped that they could see that our move to the hostel was a good one. We left Anthousa laden with toys, which Lucy quickly added to her corner of our hostel room. She was happy.

The hostel has quickly become a temporary home and our room, one of eight on the top floor, with a small balcony overlooking the main street below, our haven. That's no exaggeration. It is simply a place where both Lucy and I can relax.

We're slowly getting to know our neighbours, not easy as more often than not the children are in clinics for medication and tests or are away for a break at their real homes.

Next to the lift is petite Danae, with her two-and-a-half-year-old son Phevos, who is being treated for leukemia. Next door is Eleni with her young parents, a quiet, withdrawn couple who rarely socialise downstairs and hardly talk. Eleni is one of the few girls in Elpida who wears a wig when she ventures outside. Slightly younger then Lucy, she seems difficult and very demanding.

Next to her are Evangelitsa and her daughter Vaso, who is slightly older than Lucy. Vaso is another leukemia victim. She's been in and out of the bone marrow transplant unit and is extremely thin. She limps. No, that's wrong. It's not really a limp, she pulls one of her legs along, a problem that is more noticeable when she's tired.

Next to them and opposite us are Stella and little Panayiotis, who is nearing the end of his treatments. Stella, who seems little more than a child herself, has two older children. She is chatty, bubbly and a loving mother. Effy and Yorgos are in the far corner; Pagona, Christos and Antony are next to them; and a teenager, Vasilis, is with his parents next to us.

Lucy and I are very close with Maria, from Amaliada, and her son Nicos, who is also being treated in TAO; Smaro and Dimitri, of course; and there's also Yorgia and her daughter Maria, both tiny, with wicked laughs; Spiro, Eleni and Katerina from TAO; and two sisters, Christina and Stasa with tiny, blonde Stefanos, who are also from Rhodes.

There are others of course, parents and mothers I have met in the communal kitchen. We share thoughts and secrets as our children play together downstairs. We're all in the same boat, members of the same family, all struggling to save our children. We stay in Elpida, in hope ... where would we be without it?

On Wednesday we walked to Saint Savas from the hostel. It was quite a hike, especially for Lucy, but she managed. She was much better in the traffic and I was sure the exercise did her good. I couldn't say the same for the fresh air as I wasn't so sure that the Athens air was very fresh at all!

Both Lucy and I expected her treatment to start then, but Zampaties requested her Agia Sofia scans so we had to walk to the children's hospital. By that stage Lucy was hostile and shitty so I called Zampaties and arranged to take the scan with us on Monday. Fortunately, Smaro changed Lucy's mood, inviting us to lunch at Kolonaki where Lucy bounded about the place full of life, but Dimitri did not. Not interested in food, he was poorly, with hardly any energy at all.

If anything he seems to get his only energy from Lucy.
Is that at all possible?

In the evening, Lucy, along with Dimitri, Josef and Vaso, had an art class with an amazing woman who devoted several hours a week to the Elpida children. With endless patience and talent, she coaxed her young students to put their thoughts on paper and the colourful houses, birds and sunny landscapes they produced later decorated the playroom walls. I left Lucy in her capable hands and ran off to find a hotel room for Chris and us for the weekend. To my surprise all accommodation near the hospital and the hostel was full. I traipsed about unsuccessfully for hours and was dead tired in the evening. Lucy was a live wire.

She has amazing energy at the moment and it's nearly driving me mad. When I want to sleep, Lucy is ready to party. I'm ready to drop and she wants to draw, sing and dance, bounce on the beds, anything except sleep.
Is she scared of lying down, scared of giving in?
I can't think straight. It's 2am, my eyes want to close and all Lucy wants to do is play.

Today at Saint Savas, Zampaties and his team measured and marked Lucy's mask, explaining that the lines would ensure exact locations of the radiotherapy. It looked extremely complicated but fortunately Lucy was cooperative, joking with everyone in the room. We left the hospital laughing but, once again Lucy's mood changed dramatically. Fine one moment then she was cursing me, using the most disgusting language the next. Today she apologised and we meandered our way back to the hostel, stopping for hot chocolates and cakes on the way 'home'.

What will Lucy be like when the radiotherapy starts? What will I be like?

The Elpida staff was planning a masque party for Mardi Gras. All the children had been practising for the big night, which would run like a talent quest with, apparently, big names in Greek show business taking part. Lucy didn't want to have anything to do with it, but was coaxed into joining in by the two 'big' Dimitris (one the social worker and the other an Elpida receptionist) and smiling 'little' Dimitri, Smaro's son. She would perform a song about wearing her best party dress to a dance.

We, the parents, were to take part as well. God knows I hate things like this and usually steer well clear of anything vaguely theatrical. I was to be a bride (of all things) at a mock wedding, with Smaro as my husband. At least it was a good choice of partners!

Chris arrives tomorrow and I can't wait to see her. I desperately need to see and talk to an old friend, speak English for a while and just the thought of a change in our routine ... I can't imagine Chris' reaction when she sees us. I'm sure she'll be shocked by Lucy, or maybe not as Lucy has been amazing today, singing as if there is nothing wrong with her.

We're blessed to have a long weekend without any treatment. Seems like the timing for Chris' visit is perfectly planned.

12

Tuesday 12 March

Tuesday afternoon and I'm tired, almost numb after several extremely busy days. Lucy finally started radiation treatment yesterday, which was Monday, March 11. Her big brother's birthday.

Chris arrived on Friday afternoon. I can't explain how I feel having her here; she's like a ray of sunshine, albeit here for only a couple of days.

Chris has always been around at crucial moments of my life, ever since our crazy years together in London when I was a young travel writer and she was a pretty public relations executive. Seems like we are destined to share all the times, the good and the bad, the happy and the sad. We always talk a lot; she is a very dear friend.

She had expected to see a very changed, very ill Lucy, and while she had been quick to notice the physical changes, namely Lucy's weight loss and lack of hair, Chris was astonished at her appetite and energy level. She was also very concerned about Lucy's aggressiveness and anti-social behaviour.

She was worried about my bruised arms and worried about whether I was going to be strong enough to cope. I didn't tell her I wondered that as well.

On Friday evening we wandered the shops in the Plaka district. I was struck by the great atmosphere, the array of shops. It was fun and okay, it was carnival time. We shopped and Lucy found some cute finger puppets in a remarkable shop just off the main street. It was full of beads, baubles and quirky toys, and a goldmine of old and new treasures. We ate calamari and drank wine in a nearby taverna on one of the squares. Chris commented on Lucy's good table manners and was amazed at her appetite.

From there we wandered to Syntagma Square, which was alive with Mardi Gras celebrations courtesy of Athens' mayor. Back at the Pan Hotel, Lucy slept early, cuddled into my back as Chris and I talked into the night. We woke early and took a taxi to Agia Sofia to change the Hickman fluid. TAO was busy. Lucy and I chatted to friends and Chris was quiet, saddened, she said, by the little faces she saw.

'When I first saw Lucy I was hit by how thin she is, but in only a day I have almost forgotten that first impression. She's amazing, but now I've seen the other side because she looks just like all these little children and none of them are well, are they? God, Coll.'

Lucy wanted to go to the Acropolis, which for some reason was closed so we wandered the grounds. Lucy was fine, laughing, but suddenly turned. 'Enough of your English. I don't want to hear anymore. Enough.'

She was ghastly, spitting, cursing, beating at my already bruised arms. She wouldn't walk and demanded to be carried. Poor Chris was aghast. She kept shaking her head in disbelief.

And then Lucy stopped. As quickly as she had started she stopped and she was fine again.

Chris had to leave to catch the midday British Airways flight to London. I felt as if she was taking my happiness and liveliness with her. Her care and friendship had charged my batteries and I felt a great loss when her taxi pulled away and I had to go back into Elpida, back to what is now our real world.

A world of big questioning eyes, shiny heads and veiled thoughts.

On Sunday evening, after rehearsals for the hostel's party, Lucy was awful, shouting, crying, screaming, demanding her father. I let her cry it out and talked with Effy while Lucy played with Yorgos. We watched a very late film together.

During the weekend the weather had been wonderful, sunny and mild, but Monday morning, when we had to be at Saint Savas early, it was wild. Fortunately I managed to stop a taxi close to the hostel and we arrived at the hospital on time.

Stupidly, I hadn't asked where the treatment room was. Everyone we asked gave us different directions; one woman even told us we couldn't possibly be in the right place and tried to guide us out of the hospital again.

'This isn't a place for your child', she said. 'What on earth possessed you to bring her in here? She'll be frightened; there are too many sick, awful-looking people around. Take her out, quickly.'

I couldn't tell her why we were there, just left her shaking her head in disgust.

We found the right place in the end. The radiotherapy rooms were in the basement. I had expected one room with a waiting area but was shocked to find a number of therapy rooms off busy corridors lined with too many waiting patients.

This, sadly, was a busy place.

All eyes were on Lucy and me.

One of Zampaties' assistants appeared, smiled and knelt in front of Lucy, taking her hands and holding them in hers. 'Hi Lucy. Wow, you look pretty today. Are you ready for us? You're not nervous are you? We already know what a great little patient you are. I'll be back in a minute.'

'Lucy Mortzou.'

Hearing her name, Lucy started to sob. We stood up and I tried not to wince as she squeezed my hand so tight it hurt. A tall, blonde woman in a white medical coat reached for Lucy's other hand and we moved into the room together.

I should have noted the procedure, what the room was like, what really happened, but my only thought was Lucy. Zampaties and Thanos hurried in, made some changes to her mask and marked the base of her neck with a thick black marker pen. Lucy was lying on a bench bed with Zampaties holding the mask above her face.

'Now, Lucy, I am going to tighten this mask, it needs to be bolted to the bed so you don't move. I know that sounds scary, but trust me. I won't hurt you and you won't feel anything. Okay, Lucy? Your mother will be right outside and although you'll be alone for a few moments, we can see and hear you so don't worry.'

He touched Lucy's hand and she nodded; Lucy was okay but I felt ready to pass out.

The pretty radiologist directed me towards the door. My heart was racing. One look back at a tiny Lucy on that big bed thing and I was on the other side of the door, watching until the red light went off, signalling the end of Lucy's first radiotherapy.

She was out in minutes, thanking the staff, putting on her jacket and greeting the still-waiting older patients.

'How do you feel?'

'Fine.'

'Did it hurt?'

'No.'

'Were you scared?'

'No. Dr Zampaties said I would be fine and I was. I'm hungry though ...'

I saw no immediate side effects; in fact Lucy was brighter than ever. We even walked back to the hostel and she helped me make chocolate truffles for the evening's party.

⁓

Preparations for the talent quest followed. The lounge was decorated with streamers, balloons and paper clown's faces. A small stage was erected and seating for guests was arranged.

It was then the children's turn to get ready. Before they clambered into their Mardi Gras outfits their faces were painstakingly painted and decorated by a makeup artist who had volunteered to add her touches to the evening. Lucy's little face was covered in hearts and flowers; she twirled and laughed in her policewoman's outfit, cackling even harder as the same woman turned me into a hippy flower-power bride, complete with a long red wig. Nothing could have been more out of character. Dimitri had told me not to worry about trying to find an outfit and he had a huge grin on his face as he handed me a lacey flowery thing for my wedding dress. The sisters from Rhodes completed my outfit with high, denim platform shoes. Colleen the bride was complete.

Oh dear. The hostel quickly filled with guests, some known celebrities, pop and television stars and the wealthy ladies who support the Elpida foundation along with friends and family.

Lucy, dressed as a mini-skirted policewoman, was singing an old fashioned waltzing song to open the show. I was impressed. I had worried that she would baulk in front of so many people but she didn't, and after claiming a perfect ten from the star-studded judges' panel, she handed the stage over to Dimitri, Maria, Nicos, Antony, Maria, Katerina and many other children. Christos, a nine year-old who continued to battle his cancer and had lost his sight through his latest treatment, was outstanding, as was Layla, the little Palestinian girl who was a guest at Elpida. A reaction from her bone marrow transplant left poor Layla covered with ghastly yellow, flaky skin. She usually hid behind her mother's back and was reluctant to talk or play with the other Elpida children, but tonight she shone in a slinky outfit and a long red wig as she belted out a song by one of Greece's top female performers. Layla danced, laughed and flirted; she was a star for an evening and she won everyone's hearts.

I borrowed her wig later in my role as the blushing bride and danced with my typical sleek Greek-style 'kamaki' husband, Smaro, who was in a dark costume, sporting a moustache and a blackened front tooth, twirling large worry beads.

God, how we laughed. The party offered a chance to forget, an opportunity to dance and enjoy the music, the laughter and the feelings that abound in this special place.

We danced and sang until 1am. We cleaned and tidied until 3am but it didn't matter. We had a great night and we had laughed.

And we had forgotten.

Today (Tuesday) it seemed the hostel emptied. The girls from Rhodes, Katerina and her parents, Babis and Lucia with chubby little Yorgos, and the wonderful mother and daughter combination, Yorgia and Maria, have all gone – for the time being.

I spoke to one of the social workers about Lucy's aggressiveness and her attitude towards me. Quietly spoken Dina understood. 'I know what you are talking about. I have seen what Lucy is like. Hey, she's a wonderful little girl; everyone loves her here because she is so nice and caring. No, I mean that. She is and that's thanks to you. Lucy is a special child and if you think about it, she is only that aggressive with you.'

We talked about Lucy's upbringing, being the only girl with three older brothers, her mountain bike, the playground next to the house, athletics and swimming clubs and her boisterous friends.

Dina continued. 'You have always given her an outlet for her feelings. Now, away from all those things she has been used to, I'm afraid you're Lucy's outlet. She takes out all her feelings on you and I know that must be extremely difficult. I must add that it is better in the long run. There are other children who don't show their feelings at all, others who are aggressive all the time. We know it's difficult for you, but we [Dimitri and the rest of the staff] also know that you can cope, no matter what.'

Wednesday 13 March

Today was Lucy's third treatment, slightly later than the others and it took a long time as the machinery broke down and Lucy was moved to another room.

Strange. Lucy and I have already fallen into a new routine of arriving at the hospital, saying hello to everyone else waiting, and smiling at those who obviously didn't expect to see a child there, who were even more surprised, aghast, when she took her hat and jacket off and it was obvious that she too was awaiting treatment.

We made our way easily through the maze of hospital corridors, quickly learning the doors that opened strangely – 'No, not that one Mum, it sticks, it opens the other way' – knew exactly where to sit, where to wait, what lay in store.

Amazingly Lucy wasn't bothered by today's changes; she was taking everything in her stride. She remained calm and quiet and even said she had snoozed through the end of today's session.

After Lucy's treatment we met up with Smaro and Dimitri and decided to go to the cinema to see the new Harry Potter film. As ridiculous as it sounds, leaving the security of the hostel to venture out to the 'normal' world could be quite difficult. Both Smaro and I were having second thoughts about taking the kids out but they were adamant, so we left Elpida armed with protective green surgery masks and tissues, still wondering if we were doing the right thing.

Finding a taxi was easy as one stopped right opposite the hostel. Lucy, Dimitri and Smaro sat in the back, yours truly in the front. As soon as we took off the driver started to sneeze, the sneeze was followed quickly by a cough, then a sneezy cough. I looked back at an anxious Smaro and both children donned their masks without us saying a word.

The driver was aghast and started to cross himself, quickly, as only a good Greek Orthodox can. 'In the name of God, it's just a cold! The kids don't have to wear masks, I just have a cold!'

How could the man know that any germ could send the children into the hospital, could put them back months in their therapy?

Probably better he didn't know.

We were quickly out of the taxi (the driver, I was sure, was glad to see the back of us) and into the cinema complex. The kids were up and down the escalators, laughing at choosing huge amounts of sweets that they knew they would never eat, cackling, joking; two pairs of twinkling eyes. We paid and were directed to the door opposite the cashier. Still worrying about protecting the children, I pulled open the heavy door. The cinema was empty; we had the entire theatre to ourselves.

Dimitri and Lucy delighted in changing seats, still laughing and enjoying the movie, which took them and us out of ourselves for a couple of hours. From the cinema we wandered through a nearby park and Dimitri was suddenly tired and grouchy until we stopped for a juice and toast, which he demanded but didn't touch.

He and Lucy then found a taxi, shouting, laughing, 'Taxi, taxi, taxi!' They danced in the street, feasting on their freedom, as if they knew it might not happen again.

Friday 15 March

The fourth and fifth therapies went well, even though Lucy fretted because Zampaties was away for a few days. Thanos, the physicist, was more than willing to assist. He was full of tales of his studies in England and he wanted to impress us. He was a bit over the top but at the same time, extremely pleasant and helpful. Lucy was amazing with the other staff and I was surprised at the treatment, which seemed to have no visible side effects apart from a slight loss of appetite. She didn't vomit, wasn't dizzy, in fact we still walked to and from the hospital.

Lucy chatted easily with the hospital staff and those waiting for treatment. I suspected many looked forward to seeing her, their faces lighting up as she banged her way through the heavy entrance doors. She brightened their day. They commented on her clothes, her selection of hats, her bags and shoes, anything new. They smiled and Lucy smiled.

She no longer asked for me to be with her in the treatment room, she was confident enough by herself.

———

I have found a solution to Lucy's ongoing Hickman problem. Since the horrible rash that appeared during Lucy's chemo treatments, Lucy has been wearing a bandage to secure the Hickman pipe to her chest. Although it must have been restrictive and uncomfortable, like wearing a strapless bra, she never complained, but I knew it wasn't the perfect alternative to the sticky patch as the likelihood of infection was higher with the 'open' plug.

Last night Lucy was in Stella's room helping her with Panayiotis, when the bandage unravelled. Stella suggested trying a stretchy mesh strip, almost like a band, used by the patients in the bone marrow transplant unit and, I presumed, by burn patients who could not have adhesive tapes on their skins. Her idea was a godsend. It was much easier, less of a worry and certainly a lot more comfortable for Lucy.

After the hospital today Lucy was lost at the hostel. Dimitri and her other playmates had tests at TAO. She was difficult without company, until we were invited to a very small birthday party for Vasilis, our neighbour.

The Elpida staff that was still around late in the afternoon came upstairs for the birthday cake and Vasilis opened up to chatter. He smiled and I saw for the first time a great-looking boy.

What a shame. This bloody disease. It takes these children way too far down; down to a level I fear some never return from.

Saturday 16 March

A wonderful spring day today, as Athens, even looking from our small fifth-floor balcony, took on a totally different look. Everything seemed brighter, except for Lucy, who didn't wake until 11am. She wasn't interested in doing anything special and certainly didn't want to venture outside. She ended up making friends with Stella's older children and spent the evening with them.

Lucy is awful without company and extremely easy in it.
Her appetite has changed. She is eating less but her energy levels remain high. Every night she is a handful, bouncing about the place until way after midnight. I find it increasingly difficult and I struggle to keep my eyes open.
Closing them is not allowed. Any dozing off and Lucy is not just angry, she is bolshie and bitter. When she does finally go to sleep she sleeps like a lamb, no fighting, no snoring, no restlessness.
Guess by then she is absolutely knackered.

Sunday 17 March

My 46th birthday. My sister Jude called when I was still in bed, followed by Pat, my school friend Marg and loads of friends from Rhodes, plus I had a great text from Smaro, who was back in Thessaloniki for a few days with Dimitri. It was a good start to a very quiet birthday spent indoors with Lucy, waiting for a call from her aunt that never came.

We spent the day doing everything from cutting and pasting, embroidery and reading, to an English lesson followed by time on the laptop. Phew, I couldn't imagine what else Lucy would want to do.

Now she is playing doctors and nurses, singing to herself quite happily. What will she be like in two hours?
When she's busy and content Lucy reminds me of myself, singing and dancing to my sister's Gene Pitney records when I was about the same age. I used to hurry home from school, sneak into Jude's wardrobe and

wear her latest tartan wind jacket and high stiletto heels to swoon over *24 Hours from Tulsa*. I was content in my own world until an angry elder sister lifted the arm from the record player and whipped the jacket off my back.

Was I, as the rather spoilt youngest child of four, also such a handful, or are Lucy's mood swings just part and parcel of all this treatment?

Monday 18 March

It's Monday but there was no treatment for Lucy today as it was Clean Monday, a huge public holiday in Greece, marking the end of Mardi Gras and the beginning of 40 days' Lent. It's a day for picnicking, eating seafood and flying kites, and although Lucy waited yet again for a call from my in-laws no one phoned, so we stayed at the hostel.

Lucy wanted to eat calamari, which I found at the local market. It was good but she didn't touch it.

13

Thursday 21 March

It's the eighth day of treatment and all is going well. Lucy remains extremely active, possibly too active, too busy. The only side effect of the treatment appears to be a change in appetite. She is eating less but still eating.

The Saint Savas routine continued. Lucy had got to know all the regulars there. One of her favorites was a lovely quiet woman called Voula, who was recovering from breast cancer. Petite and well dressed with light brown, shoulder length hair, she looked particularly good today and I told her so. Tears started to stream down her cheeks.

'I'm having a bad day today. I woke feeling down and nothing seems right.'

'Come on,' I persisted, 'you look fine. Heavens, I would give anything to have your hair, it always looks so good.'

'So it should, I paid enough for it,' she said, lifting a perfectly fitted wig slightly off her head. I was speechless. How could I have been so stupid? Voula laughed.

'Oh, your face, Colleen! It's a picture. Hey, don't worry about it; at least you made me laugh!'

I hugged her and believed she needed it. Didn't we all.

Many of the regulars weren't there today and Thanos was helping.

He had the ability to make the patients feel special, was especially good with Lucy and went out of his way to brighten her day. He always talked to me in English, and was obviously concerned about Lucy and our future. He asked why we were always alone and noted the lack of support from anyone else in the family. I told him quickly that the boys were on Rhodes, that I was going through a separation, and that it was difficult.

'Things will get better,' he said. 'You are about the most positive person I have come across in this hospital. You believe that Lucy will get well and that shows in your daughter as well. She's very ill but she's a fighter and although her case is a particularly difficult one, I'm pretty sure she will make it. With your support of course.'

For a physicist he was pretty good at psychology.

Katerina was there today. At 27 (Lucy asked her age) she was the youngest of the trio. She wore New Age-type clothes and seemed older than her years, but was obviously very good and dedicated to her work.

A threesome also ran the radiotherapy control room. Rea reigned supreme as chief technologist. Short-haired, tall, boyish and bossy, Rea took no nonsense as she moved about on absurdly high heels. Her assistant, Penny, was tall and attractive, with amazing hair and makeup, her bright clothing a rainbow of colours in the drab radiation room. She was pretty, chatty and unruffled. Anastasia was the most natural of the three women, with an open, easy smile and nondescript clothing. She wore clogs or runners.

And the regulars? Well, of course there was Voula, who was around my age, twice married. She told me that her second husband left her just as her treatment started and she had lost her breast. Nice.

Eve was middle-aged, friendly, and always greeted Lucy, although Lucy didn't always respond. She bought a Barbie doll for Lucy at the end of her treatment; she bought one for Vaso too, because she thought she might need one. Another woman, whose name I don't know, gave Lucy a light green trouser and sleeveless jacket suit. 'Just a little something for her to wear at Easter,' she explained.

They were all kind, supportive people. An elderly nun who was always accompanied by another little nun gave Lucy a beautiful little cross, made out of pearls.

This evening Lucy and I went shopping, a mini expedition from the hostel, with Effy and Yorgos and Stella and little Panayiotis in a pushchair. With Panayiotis nearing the end of his treatment Stella was looking for gifts for his doctors and nurses. She was, it seemed, intent on trying every perfume and cologne in the beauty shop. Stella sprayed the perfumes, keeping her masked baby away from the smells, trying to get us involved. We were doing our best to keep Yorgos and Lucy from touching everything in sight. It was a circus, the beauty department was turned upside down and even I ended up buying some makeup.

The main thing was that we didn't stop laughing.

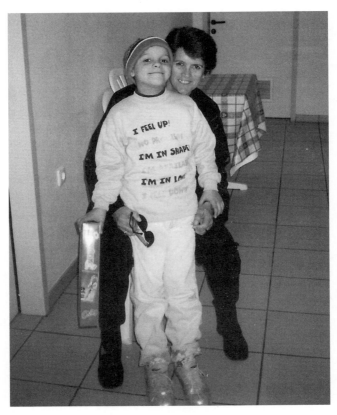

In the corridor outside our room at Elpida hostel:
we had just returned from a radiotherapy session at
Agios Savas with Lucy holding one of the many gifts
she received from other outpatients there

Friday 22 March

Up early and off to Saint Savas by 10.30. The ninth session today and somehow there was a change in Lucy. She didn't want breakfast and was tired and complained of aches after the treatment. We had to go to TAO to change the Hickman fluid, and also to check on a cough she'd developed that had others in the hostel, ever conscious of infections and germs, eyeing her suspiciously. Even Stella had asked her to wear a mask when she was near Panayiotis.

We stopped twice walking from one hospital to the other, but Lucy seemed happier and livelier when Papadakis explained that she didn't have a cold, that the cough could be regarded as a normal side effect.

Like all the other children, Lucy has gotten used to wearing the light green masks, a precaution if there are any germs about. She wears one whenever we go into Saint Savas and quickly pulls it off outside, unless it is a particularly smoggy Athens morning. Lucy isn't used to wearing a mask at the hostel and she didn't like the thought that some of the parents were worried about her cough.

Wednesday 27 March

It's Wednesday evening, just after a small celebration for Independence Day, which was actually two days ago. The hostel had the kids' celebration tonight ... a mini parade with flags and short speeches in the playroom.

The Elpida staff ensure that birthdays, name days and public holidays are celebrated. It's important that daily life in the hostel resembles the children's daily lives outside.

On Saturday afternoon Maria called and invited us over for the long weekend. I was surprised and Lucy was delighted. Within an hour we were on the bus to Anthousa. We did little there but it was pleasant, although Lucy was troubled by the cough that by Monday evening sounded awful.

After her tenth treatment yesterday we went straight to TAO, concerned about the cough and the possibility that it was a dreaded cold. Her doctor said no but prescribed a cough medicine and warned Lucy that her throat would feel sore and raw. He wasn't particularly worried. I tried to imagine what her throat might look like after the chemo and the ongoing radiotherapy. The cough apart, Lucy showed no other side effects and externally there was no difference to her face or skin.

In the evening we waited to see Smaro and Dimitri but they arrived back at TAO late, too late even for Lucy.

Stupid me, I am writing away and somehow forgetting the highlight of the afternoon. Lucy had another visit from the Make A Wish volunteers.

I sat in the dining room chatting with Maro and Lucy was in the lounge for a long time with Mari. After what seemed an age, Mari joined us. She had a strange look on her face. She was smiling but her eyes were brimming with tears.

My first thought was that Lucy had lost her temper and showed someone the side she kept only for me. I felt myself taking a deep breath as Mari reached for my hand.

'You have a very special little girl there, Colleen.' I relaxed but then realised she was ready to cry.

'Lucy told me she has given a lot of thought to her wish. And she has because she mentioned a lot of wishes we have granted to other children.' She paused to wipe her eyes. 'Do you know what she wants to do? She wants to go to New Zealand to see her Nana – that's right isn't it? That's how she calls her grandmother there?'

'Lucy wants to go to New Zealand and she wants her brothers to go with her.' Mari was still threatening to cry, but she smiled as Lucy joined us.

'Leave it to us Lucy. If you want to see your Nana then you'll see your Nana. We'll be in touch,' she said as the two women made their way towards the lift.

I was flabbergasted.

'How did you think of that? I thought you wanted to go to Disneyland or somewhere like that.'

'I don't know, Mum. It just came and then I thought it would be awful to leave my brothers behind, so I asked if they could come too ...'

Lucy knows Mum only as a voice at the end of the telephone at Christmas and on special occasions. Of course she's seen her in photos but doesn't remember meeting her as Mum's last visit to Greece was for Lucy's christening.
Just imagine going home ...
Lucy will have to get better first.
Heavens, my heart is racing for a happy reason this time.

Today (Tuesday) we went to Saint Savas with Smaro and Dimitri, who needed some radiotherapy before going into the bone marrow transplant unit. Smaro told me how his specialists had struggled to find a suitable bone marrow donor and how they had found a match in a gentleman from Cyprus. The sooner the treatments began, the sooner the transplant could go ahead and the sooner Dimitri would be well again.

Lucy's treatment was very quick and we waited as preparations were made for Dimitri's five full-body treatments.

From there we all went to TAO, where Lucy's doctor once again checked her cough, which has definitely worsened. He confirmed it was a result of the treatment, adding that, unfortunately, it would probably get worse! The only positive news was that is was nothing that the other children could catch.

'Huh,' Lucy said. 'Try telling that to the mothers in Elpida, and in the waiting room here. They all gave me awful looks when I coughed, didn't they Mum? I told them I haven't got a cold but I know they don't believe me.' Dr Papadakis smiled at his tough little patient.

'That's okay Lucy. We know you haven't got a cold and that you aren't spreading germs. But just to be safe and to stop all those gossiping mothers out there, I suggest you wear a mask for a few days. Okay?'

So Lucy wore her mask constantly. She was not happy about it but she did as her doctor said.

Thursday 28 March

Twelfth treatment today and Lucy was tired and irritable afterwards. She didn't eat at all in the morning and was much, much slower walking to the hospital.

Cecilia had called so following the treatment we took the Metro downtown and had lunch at her apartment. Much to everyone's surprise Lucy ate pork chops and chips, olives and cucumber. In fact she asked for more cucumber and had Cecilia and her husband Panayiotis in fits of laughter. Lucy was in good form and when we left late in the afternoon she had me crying with laughter on the bus ride home.

For some reason the bus rolled, or seemed to, and Lucy found it very funny. We giggled all the way until the bus stopped outside the Elpida gate. Lucy was just in time for music and games with her friends.

Friday 29 March

The thirteenth treatment – and the final for the week – and Voula invited us for lunch on Sunday.

Lucy's cough was worse. She refused to take the prescribed cough medicine and antibiotics. Ah, she was an angel in front of her doctor, quiet, cooperative. 'Yes, sure, I will take the medicine.'

That was until we were back at the hotel where she threw the bottles into the cupboard. 'Leave them there. Leave them in the cupboard where I have put them,' she screamed.

She was stubborn and refused to budge. I told her that her cough would get worse. I might as well have talked to the wall.

In the afternoon Effy decided we should go for a drive. She had her Suzuki jeep in Athens so, armed with a map and me as co-driver, we headed off towards the harbour area of Piraeus. When I said left, she went right; when I suggested we turn a corner, she continued straight ahead. Eventually we found the coastline and stopped at Microlimano. It was bliss to be the near the sea again, laughing with the kids, who had a wonderful time with hot chocolates and little biscuits and cocktail goodies. We laughed and sang in the car, getting lost in the maze of

Athens' streets. It didn't matter. Once again, laughter was proving to be the best medicine.

Saturday 30 March

We tried the same formula today and found the aptly named Up Down coffee shop, but it wasn't quite the same. Still, Lucy and Yorgos, who was undergoing intermittent chemotherapy, were at least out of their everyday routines.

Sunday 31 March

Lucy and I were to go to Voula's house for lunch today, but it was not to be. As soon as she opened her eyes Lucy was adamant that we were not going anywhere. Her stubbornness and moodiness magnified, and as was so often the case, there was no way of changing her mind.

I gave up and settled in to watch television, feeling too bruised mentally and physically (Lucy was unusually strong and nasty today) to tackle anything else.

However, Effy had other plans for us. She'd heard our argument and came up with a solution in the form of her friend Lucas, who took us with them on a Sunday drive out of Athens and along the coast. A fast BMW, good music and a good-looking young man who had Lucy blushing every time he spoke to her ...

Thanks Effy!
What a strange time ... hospitals, treatments, masks, sick people, the hostel, friends, nerves, stress ... escape.

Monday 1 April
– April Fool's Day

I lie in bed waiting for Lucy to wake, and think about April Fool's Day. It's an apt name. Are we, all of us in the hostel, in the clinic, are we all fools living in hope of cures, looking forward to the end of the treatments, time with our families, a normal life again?

Our children are all on the same path, similar treatments, experiencing the same pains and problems and we are all hoping there is a light at the end of the tunnel.

Is there? Or are we fools to continue hoping?

Fourteenth treatment today and Lucy was all apologies to Voula. With raw nerves and still feeling bruised, I opted to stay away from chatting. All the Agios Savas patients waited for Lucy to brighten their day; she was their ray of sunshine, their little ray of hope, and I didn't want anything I said to ruin that. We just said she hadn't felt so good and that was that.

Dimitri started his treatment day with a long, three-hour session, where he was moved and re-positioned constantly. It must be incredibly tiring for such a little body. He was exhausted and went straight back to the hostel.

Lucy and I had checked in at TAO first. Her blood tests were good and they said her cough, definitely from the treatment, was nothing to worry about.

Are they joking?

We returned to the hostel to bad news. Our neighbour, Vasilis, had died. Our safe little world was blown apart. I'd heard that he had been readmitted to hospital but didn't realise he was so sick again. Vasilis was 14. He'd been through a successful bone marrow transplant and a sudden reaction to it had turned him into a wheelchair-bound monster, a figure from which most of the children in the hostel hurried away.

Some days pass here so easily, so pleasantly, that I forget – for a while – why Lucy is here. She doesn't have any noticeable side effects. Apart from her hair, which is now growing back, she looks as good if not better than before.

But what happened to Vasilis? He was a fine-looking boy, ready to tackle anything, smiling his way into manhood. I wonder if the same could happen to Lucy.

No. Lucy can only get better.

For me there is no alternative.

One moment we were mourning, the next we were looking forward to a treat. We were whisked off to a theatre, to a one-off production, supported by the Elpida Foundation. Dimitri had kept the news of the outing as a surprise. It was perfectly timed to lift our lagging spirits.

It wasn't easy to get an unannounced outing ready for 'takeoff' but Dimitri and his assistants managed to have the Elpida parents and children (plus Alexandros and Joanna, who were visiting) on the coach, being transported through the city, on time.

We looked like any other coach full of young kids on a school outing, only most of the Elpida children were wearing surgical masks; the clamour, noise and excitement were the same. The production was aptly named Ενα αλλιώτικο ταξιδι, *A Special Trip, A Journey with a Difference.* It was staged by known actors and children suffering from Down's syndrome and other physical and mental disabilities.

At the theatre we were introduced to Marianna Vardinoyanni, the amazing woman who is president of the Elpida Foundation. A quietly spoken and elegant lady, she welcomed the TAO children with open arms, greeting them and us (the mothers) as if we were old friends. In the theatre we had allotted seats and the two rows in front of and behind us were to remain empty. The children from Elpida, it seemed, needed their germ-free space, for a while at least, until the huge theatre filled with celebrities, the ex-prime minister's wife and children with special needs.

When the production started there was complete and utter silence. The youngsters forgot their tiredness, any whining stopped; nothing, it seemed, could distract their attention.

Afterwards we returned to the hostel boosted in a way by the fine performance and, in another, subdued.

Why does Lucy have to go through all of this?

Why can't she just have a normal life like all of her noisy, giggly little girlfriends in Rhodes? Why, why, why?

Why are we here in Athens? Why Lucy? Why did Vasilis and Pandelis have to die? Why do these other remarkable children have to go through life marked by their disabilities?

Why?

Tuesday 2 April

Number fifteen today. We are nearing the turning point. Lucy wasn't good early this morning. She wasn't feeling well and although she was grumpy we didn't argue. Poor Dimitri suffered badly through his treatments. He was exhausted and vomiting while Lucy, thank God, had just the cough and, of course, her nerves.

Again I wondered if Lucy was going to make it. Would she beat this illness? I had to keep telling myself the only answer was YES.

Wednesday 10 April

I have more than a week to catch up in this notebook. A week of ups and downs, treatments, tantrums, tears and laughter. Sometimes in the middle of the night, when I am fighting to find sleep, my head fills with thoughts, emotions, feelings that I should write down. Most of them, however, are negative.

I feel we are surrounded by death. It's like a shroud, a cover that lifts and hovers. Lucy is dicing with death, living and gambling with it and I wonder if she is going to beat it in the end.

I think of it every day as we walk towards Saint Savas. The walks are slower, more difficult, but she still manages. The sirens of the ambulances that scream through the Athens traffic freeze my soul and I wonder why. We have never been in an ambulance but each time I see or hear one I wonder whose turn it is.

I want to cry and often the tears fall almost unnoticed. Is there a child inside, being rushed to the hospital? Is it an older person being taken somewhere else? Does it really matter if they are young or old? We, no matter what age we are, are just older children, but somehow seeing a child suffer is worse.

The sirens really bother me. It's a morbid straight-to-the-stomach feeling that I can't control. I wonder why this is happening to me now as I wasn't bothered before. It's almost like panic.

Maybe it has something to do with marks that have appeared on Lucy's face. This heavy radiation treatment is leaving its signs.

Since the weekend Lucy had marks, like burn marks, above her cheekbones, and now all over her neck and lower cheeks. She looked like she had been in the sun too long.

Zampaties saw it today and said there was nothing to worry about. I hoped he was right. It was difficult, different, suddenly seeing signs of the treatment. Lucy's appetite also changed dramatically. She picked at her food with little interest. Her temperament, however, was much improved and she was sleeping earlier and longer.

Little Dimitri had moved from TAO into the Transplant unit and, after the bone marrow transplant, will be in isolation for at least one month.

Lucy will miss his company and I will miss his wonderful, wide smile. Ready to leave the hostel last Friday, he came up to the fifth floor to say goodbye to Lucy, who had been reluctant to go and see him off.

'Bye Lucy,' he said from behind the green mask, which seemed to dwarf his little face. 'You'll wait for me, won't you?'

'Of course I will!'

Their farewell was touching, almost formal, and I couldn't look at Smaro as she moved away, not daring to say anything through quivering lips. They hugged and little Dimitri left and I felt dreadful.

Tuesday's treatment was routine and we were back at the hostel early to wait for a visitor. John Nightingale is a friend of mine from Lindos. He had been one of our first 'learners' when Yorgos and I had started up our water ski business a month after getting married. John used to sail into Lindos Bay with friends from England every summer. They were all single men, intent on taking Lindos by storm, and that they did most evenings. John rarely managed to finish his cheap-rate block of skiing lessons. He did, however, learn to monoski (on the bet of a bottle of champagne that I still owed him) and went on to establish his own water ski school in Lindos after Yorgos and I decided to live in Rhodes town.

John had called to say he was passing through Athens en route to Rhodes for the coming summer season. 'Could we meet up?'

Why not? He was a good friend. I jumped at the opportunity to speak English and Lucy brightened at the thought of eating out. She chose the venue: Goody's Fast Food, which was just a few minutes' walk from the hostel. We invited Effy and Yorgos to join us. John joined us later for a special mid-afternoon service at the hostel. I smiled at the questioning faces of the Elpida staff. They saw Lucy was relaxed and happy with this unknown Englishman. I could read their thoughts, 'Mmmm, who is this man with Colleen?'

I left them to wonder as the priest ploughed through an extremely long blessing that sent the usually restless and mischievous Josef to sleep and had Lucy very nearly setting the Elpida lounge on fire with the candles. John kept moving his head, eyes squinting; he was impressed, although we were all a bit fidgety by the end of it. It was during the service that Dimitri caught my eye and, looking at Lucy, put his hands to his face and neck; like me he was concerned about the marks that were becoming more noticeable.

John and I went for a drink and sat for an hour in a local coffee shop afterwards. He was, as always, slightly flirtatious, good company; he was also very worried about my daughter.

The next day I made sure the Saint Savas doctors looked at Lucy's skin. Zampaties prescribed two ointments, which had to be used simultaneously. As usual I had to run to the IKA hospital to get it checked by the doctors there and then find a pharmacy that had the special creams. They were extremely expensive but I didn't care, as long as they stopped the burning on Lucy's face.

Thursday 18 April

Many days have passed. We have been busy, busy doing nothing I guess. Lucy is nearing the end of radiotherapy and isn't at her best. Her neck is burned and marked; she has virtually lost her voice and suffers with terrible phlegm. No one warned me of these side effects. I'm scared but, as always, try not to show it.

Until now no one, apart from those who know what type of cancer Lucy is fighting, has really taken any notice of her physical condition. She's always pleasant with people, easy to get on with and, of course, terribly cute. Now that there's evidence that she is having treatment people are somehow treating her differently; you can see in their faces that they feel sorry for her.

The nights are difficult. Lucy is snoring again. She's restless, sleeps fitfully and wakes many times during the night to clear her throat. Last night she bolted upright in bed, with no idea where she was or what she was doing. Her cough was choking and the sheets were full of phlegm and blood. It was a terrible mess. I quickly changed the sheets and, thankfully, a dazed and exhausted Lucy went straight back to sleep.

I was shaking from fright and didn't sleep again.

I feel we are going backwards instead of making any progress. I'm trying not to pass my fears on to Lucy but that's not easy when we are all day, every day together.

Her hair is growing back but she still dislikes going anywhere without a hat. She is also wearing a mask most times when we go out and always at the hospital. She knows when she needs it. She knows best.

Yesterday Zampaties and his team altered her mask to minimise the treatment on the badly burned neck area. Zampaties has been strange and hasn't helped my anguish over Lucy's appearance.

'You know we are doing all we can for Lucy', he said, as if she was into her last days and something was going wrong. I noticed he looked at her sometimes as if he was hurting. Yesterday he admitted he wasn't sleeping well. 'I keep thinking about your Lucy, our Lucy. We all try not to get emotionally attached to our patients because that makes our work so difficult, but that's impossible with Lucy. We all love her.' He paused, running his hand through his wild hair slowly to scratch the back of his head. 'My daughter is the same age as Lucy. I just can't imagine how I would feel, how I would react were she that ill.'

He touched my shoulder and walked away, leaving me to wonder whether all this treatment was working or not.

―

Last week we visited Agia Sofia's other cancer clinic, the one Lucy was to go to originally. Yorgos was a KETH patient and needed to see his specialist in the evening; Effy wanted company and Lucy was inquisitive.

'Let's go and see what KETH is like, Mum,' she urged. I wasn't keen. I didn't need to be reminded of that awful day that had changed our lives, but Lucy was persuasive.

We sat in the waiting room while Effy and Yorgos waited for his doctor. The clinic seemed oppressive, cold and deadly quiet, the empty waiting room leading to a corridor of closed doors. Yorgos' specialist was not there so we took a taxi to her surgery, a five-minute drive from the hospital. Queuing for a bus back to the hostel, the children, who were both wearing masks, caught the attention of a well-coiffed middle-aged woman. Looking aghast, she turned to Effy and launched into a startling diatribe. 'Why in God's name are your children wearing masks? I just can't believe the things that you trendy mothers will do … there's nothing wrong with the air here in Athens. Good grief, putting them in those masks makes them look hideous, like cancer kids or something.'

Effy, never one to mince words went to say something but she wasn't quick enough. The woman continued. 'There is nothing I hate more than over-protective parents. I'm a psychologist and a social worker and I don't often give free advice but let me tell you you're doing your children nothing but harm making them wear masks.'

Effy was ropeable. 'If you are so well educated and knowledgeable, you silly cow, you should know better than to stare so openly at our children.'

Oops. I could feel it getting nasty and flagged down a taxi. The kids were quick to jump in and, as if on cue, pulled off their hats and their masks and waved at the woman. Her horrified face had them both in fits. I thanked God that we got away from a full-scale argument and that the children had added their touch to the scene. I did wonder later though if that woman had a flourishing business. I hoped not, having heard what kind of advice she could give.

Wednesday 24 April

I should be writing every day but more often than not I am tired, drained and my whole body aches. I even slept for a couple of hours yesterday afternoon, which is something I never do.

Neither Lucy nor I are sleeping properly. Her nose is stuffed, she snores and she wakes often in coughing fits to clear her throat of the bloody phlegm that is choking her system. A couple of times I've been ready to rush her into the clinic but she vomits up the phlegm and relaxes immediately. I lie watching her sleep, hoping and praying it won't happen again. Her doctors tell me that the phlegm is an expected side effect of the treatment. I just wish they'd told me earlier and I could have been a little more prepared.

Lucy's voice has also changed drastically, from croaky over the past few days to virtually non-existent. The doctors tell me don't panic, everything will return to normal.

Will it? Ever?

I booked flights to Rhodes for Easter. Lucy and I were both looking forward to the break but I was worried about her voice. Another problem was a flu epidemic that was closing schools throughout Greece.

Was it a good idea to travel?

Lucy would have to wear a mask at Yorgos' workshop, near any animals and, now, near any other adults or children. Lucy donned the mask very easily in Athens, but would she do the same in Rhodes?

On Saturday Lucy and I revisited Saint Ephraim, this time with Effy and Yorgos. Lucy was very happy to be going back to the monastery; she had become one of the saint's biggest fans. The drive was full of chat and laughter. We sang most of the way, adding our own touches to the songs offered by the local radio station. In high spirits we laughed our way into the monastery courtyard, where we were directed by a disapproving nun into a small room packed with flowing skirts and loose blouses. The nun didn't disapprove of our smiles; it was Effy's rather tight top that did not go down well. More laughter as she redressed and we moved into the church.

I was thinking about my first visit, the changes in Lucy and her belief in the saint's powers. She caught my brimming eyes as I fought back the tears. 'Must be an allergy to whatever incense they are burning in here,' I told her. Lucy would have believed my white lie had she not noticed the tears streaking Effy's face too.

Effy was a different person for a while, distant, in another world, thinking and praying. She remained reserved until we settled to eat at a restaurant on the seafront. We watched Yorgos and Lucy playing on the playground swings, not a care in the world. On our return to Elpida, Effy was still unusually quiet and she obviously didn't want to talk about whatever was on her mind.

15

Friday 25 April

Today marked the end of Lucy's radiation treatment and heavens – what a relief.

The previous few days had been difficult. Tired, lethargic, with little to say to the other patients and the Agios Savas staff, Lucy was tearful before going into the treatment room. She'd had enough, physically and mentally. The strain on her frail little body was showing, not just in the burns, which were not as raw now, but also in the daily blood tests that Agios Savas requested to ensure that she was strong enough to cope with the treatments. For the first time Lucy was on the borderline.

This morning, however, Lucy smiled when I woke her.

'It's my last one today, eh Mum?'

I didn't have to ask her to do anything. She was ready before I was, rushing out the door towards the lift. I'd already told her I would buy treats for the Agios Savas staff and she pulled me into the corner cake shop. She did the talking and she chose the cakes. She was happy and it showed. Laden down with boxes of cakes, we took a taxi to the hospital. Lucy was a different child, bounding along the hospital corridors and downstairs to the radiology department. She offered everyone cakes, had the cheekiest of grins for Zampaties and Thanos, and her final therapy was over in a smile as Lucy walked away from Agios Savas, her hands full of gifts from patients and the doctors and their assistants.

Unlike Agia Sofia, Agios Savas did not offer automatic national insurance payments. I had to pay in cash and was told that a full refund would be arranged from my local IKA office on Rhodes. I took the necessary papers and, with Lucy, walked through the entrance gates with mixed feelings. It was rather like leaving TAO for the first time; I felt somewhat unsure of the future. Yes, Lucy had finished her harsh treatments, but now a waiting game began. We waited to see if the treatments had been successful. Later, scans would show the results. We could only be patient.

That evening we met with her TAO specialist again. 'The worst is over for Lucy,' he said. 'I know it's been difficult seeing the physical signs of her illness; I realise she still has the problem with the phlegm and the changes in her voice, but be patient. Lucy is a fighter; she's amazed everyone with her spirit. She's beating this, I am sure.'

He spoke a little about Lucy's next treatment, explaining it would involve six months of immunotherapy with interferon injections that would, hopefully, stop any cancerous cells from growing. 'This is something new for us. This drug has not been used as part of treatment for a child suffering from cancer in Greece,' he said, showing me emails and correspondence with cancer specialists from Germany. 'Lucy shouldn't suffer many side effects. We'll need to keep a careful watch at first of course, but I am sure, all going well, after a month or so you will be able to return home and continue the treatment on Rhodes.' Turning to Lucy, who had been telling him her plans for Easter on Rhodes, Papadakis said, 'Okay, little Miss Rhodes, I want you to be a complete snob there, big sun hat, Barbie glasses, show those local boys what you have learned during your stay in Athens.'

Lucy laughed, not realising that the hats and glasses were a necessity after her treatments: 'If I have to wear them, then Mum has to buy them, isn't that right?' Papadakis grinned.

'Go on, get out of here,' he said to Lucy. 'Oops, sorry about that,' he added, holding the door open for me. 'Happy shopping and Happy Easter. Relax a little, she's looking good.'

Of course we stopped at the opticians on the road back to Elpida, and of course Lucy chose a pair of sunglasses. The frames were bright pink and matched the paler pink sun hat we purchased further along the block.

Later in the evening I sat out on the balcony with Effy while Lucy and Yorgos were in the hostel playroom. She was drinking a Baileys and I had poured a small whisky; neither was really allowed in the hostel but we had cause to celebrate, and Effy needed to talk. I had noticed that Yorgos was having more tests than usual but Effy hadn't said anything and I hadn't pried, knowing that she would tell me what was on her mind when she was ready to.

Flushed with the Baileys, Effy started to explain. 'Yorgos' treatments had been going as planned until a month ago when a scan showed fluid around his remaining kidney. It wasn't just that there was some fluid, there was too much.'

His specialist, my dreaded woman in green, had advised a series of ultrasounds, every second day for a month, to monitor the state of the fluid. Effy and Yorgos had gone to the hospital every second day for an ultrasound, until the doctor decided to get a second opinion. She wanted ultrasounds from a private clinic.

'I was shattered. I appreciated the fact that she wanted another opinion but, as you know only too well, life's difficult enough at the moment without having to go private. I knew I couldn't afford to go out of the hospital to have the ultrasounds so I told her I didn't have the extra money to pay for those tests. She gave me an address and told me not to worry about payment, she would take care of that, and so the ultrasounds continued privately. I didn't pay. Yorgos' specialist knew I couldn't pay but they did the ultrasounds anyway and each one showed the same thing, fluid around his one good, functioning kidney.

'The Friday before the final ultrasound we had yet another appointment with his specialist. She was blunt, as always, and told me that if it didn't show any change, if the fluid hadn't moved, if it was still the same, she was afraid that we would have to stop all treatment.

'She told me that Yorgos' body wouldn't be able to cope with any more chemotherapy.'

Wiping away a stream of tears, Effy continued, 'I felt that it was the end for us, that whatever Yorgos had gone through until then amounted to nothing. We had one last chance; that was it.'

That was before the weekend we had visited Agios Ephraim.

'I prayed to the saint to help Yorgos. I prayed like I have never prayed before. I asked him to help. Yorgos desperately needed it, I needed it.

'When we came back to the hostel that evening I couldn't let him out of my sight. I knew Agios Ephraim would help us. I kept telling myself that there was no way that Yorgos wouldn't finish his treatment. I didn't sleep at all, just watched him and willed his body to get rid of the fluid. I wanted to draw it off with a syringe; I was so desperate to do something. The only good thing was that I felt so positive that night.

'The next day Yorgos had his final ultrasound. When he had finished, the technician looked bewildered.

'When he handed me the results he had the strangest look on his face; he looked like he couldn't believe what he was seeing. He didn't make any comment, just told us to go straight to the clinic. Well, you can imagine how I felt. I rushed Yorgos back to KETH where his doctor had that same unbelieving look. She told me she was amazed, that the fluid had gone, it was hardly visible and that Yorgos' treatments could continue.

'We came back to Elpida, I made myself a stronger than normal coffee [Effy's "normal" coffee was lethal] and I thought, "Hey, we're back in the game."'

Effy paused and we both took long sips of our drinks, not saying anything for a long time. Then I hugged her and we had another drink.

Wednesday 1 May

We are ready to leave for Rhodes for Easter. Lucy is at the computer playing a card game, killing time until the taxi arrives to take us to the airport. She can't wait to leave. I feel drained, tired, and uncertain.

Panayiota and little Elena are struggling. I pray they'll be okay, that they will find strength from somewhere, but hey, they've struggled for so long, battling an enemy who is closing in, sensing victory.

Saturday 11 May

It's Saturday afternoon and we're back in the hostel. The local church, Saint Thomas, is celebrating its Name Day and the entire road from the hospital to the hostel is like a huge market, with everything from honey balls and candyfloss to shoes, goldfish and CDs for sale. Looking down from our balcony the view is amazing, a vast array of underwear, sexy thongs, frilly knickers, tiny and humongous bras. Lucy and I have been out twice but it's an expensive venture; it's hard to walk by the stalls, all so colourful and lively, and we've both found little trinkets and bargains.

Lucy's fine, recharged from a week in Rhodes where, as always, she spent most of her time with her father, grandmother and friends.

I had a feeling that Rhodes would be difficult for me this time and it was. The house was dirty and untidy but, knocked by a bout of flu, I did nothing for the first three days. I suffered a sore, burning throat, had no appetite and little or no voice; a tiny taste of what Lucy has been going through. I suffered those symptoms for three days and still feel weakened by the bug. How had Lucy managed? Mine was nothing, just a cold; Lucy had been to hell and back and she was still fighting.

On Rhodes I explained to everyone, father and grandmother in particular, that Lucy had to be careful and would be a bit of a worry in the evenings as she was still throwing up phlegm. I think they thought I was over-reacting as for the first couple of days they said she slept well.

Then the shock came!

Lucy must have been very tired and had a difficult night, coughing and choking until she vomited the bloody phlegm that continued to clog her throat. Yorgos panicked and was ready to take her to the hospital, but after clearing her throat, Lucy relaxed and slept again.

Awful to admit but I was glad they experienced that and saw I wasn't being excessive. I was being careful and realistic. I also warned that she shouldn't be near animals and that her doctors had said she could play with friends but had to stay away from draughts and strong winds. Motorbikes were definitely out.

Speaking to the deaf or the dead would have had a greater effect.

On Easter Sunday her father had a barbecue. When I pulled up outside the workshop he was spit roasting a lamb or goat in a field opposite his fibreglass boat-building yard. There were pigs running wild, cows to the side, dogs barking, and moulds of fibreglass boats everywhere, including some that had been upturned to serve as feeding troughs for the animals.

I was revolted by the whole thing, the workshop and the muck and filth around it, and wondered how he made any money.
I digress.

Looking slightly beyond the chaos, my next view was of Lucy, clinging to her brother on the back of a small motorbike. She was on the bike just long enough to tear a chunk of skin from her heel.

She was upset. 'You won't tell my doctor, will you Mum?' I was livid, but not with her or with my smiling son who thought he was doing Lucy a special favour. I was livid, smack in the face angry, with my husband.

'You really have no idea what this is all about do you?' I cried. 'You haven't seen what tricks cancer has up its sleeve. You can't gamble with this sickness, you just can't. For God's sake, look after your daughter!'

I felt sick and wanted to leave. Lucy would not join me. She sat close to her father and ignored me.

'Listen, I'm sorry,' Yorgos said. 'We'll be more careful.'

I left and hurried home to collapse, a sniffling, coughing wreck, on my couch. I was aching, tired, angry and ill. I felt empty and I didn't want anything.

And then the worst happened.

My mobile buzzed and it was Smaro. She was upset and crying and could barely talk.

'It's Panayiota.'

A long pause and a heavy sigh. 'Oh Colleen, our brave little friend has died.' Although we all knew there was little or no hope for Panayiota, the news of her death was a shock, a slap in the face.

I can't stop the tears. Panayiota had told me she felt jealous of Lucy at the beginning, jealous of her long blonde hair, her looks, her liveliness; she had sobbed when Lucy lost her hair and she knew that they were fighting the same enemy. Panayiota was a young girl who didn't have a chance to live, a chance to love.

Goodbye Panayiota. I will try to remember you smiling.

Rhodes should have been a pleasant break but somehow it wasn't. I spent great moments with the boys, teaching the twins to drive, laughing in the bowling alley when my luck was running and they and their friends thought I was an expert. I spent a lot of time walking on the beach, feeling I couldn't get enough of the fresh air and the sea.

Truth is I couldn't get enough. I wanted our normal life back, I wanted my boys, I wanted Lucy to laugh and smile. I wanted her well again.

16

Sunday 12 May

Mother's Day today. I called Mum, who sounded great. She was happy to hear from me and to learn about Lucy's progress. Of course I didn't go into too many details, just said she was fine and, I added casually, looking forward to seeing her soon.

'Wouldn't that be wonderful dear? Imagine Lucy coming here and meeting all the lovely people that have been praying her for so long. I'll get Pat to buy a Lotto ticket and if I win I'll get you and the children over here as soon as Lucy is well enough. That would be nice, wouldn't it dear?'

I'd not mentioned anything to Mum about Lucy's wish, as I was reluctant to tell her that Make A Wish could be arranging a trip to Christchurch. I didn't want her getting her hopes up to be disappointed if the trip was not approved.

But it was Mother's Day so I just suggested that we could be seeing her.

'Well that's something else that I can get my friends to pray for!' Mum said.

Her response to my news was quick and very typical May Morgan logic.

Lucy and I have settled back into the everyday life at Elpida, checking at TAO every few days for blood tests and to change the Hickman fluid. Her facial burns are lighter, she looks badly sunburnt, and her voice is slowly returning to normal. Our nights are no longer interrupted with her coughing and choking.

Her specialist remains confident and, with her blood test results showing improvements, says she is close to starting her immunotherapy. This time I feel I am a step ahead of her treatment as I have used some of my quieter hours to learn more about it through the Internet. As always, the online information is very detailed, much of it using medical terms I don't understand.

MedicineNet.com defines immunology as a treatment:

---

to stimulate or restore the ability of the immune (defense) system to fight infection and disease.

Immunotherapy (also called biological therapy or biotherapy) often employs substances called biological response modifiers (BRMs). The body normally produces low levels of BRMs in response to infection and disease. Large amounts of BRMs can be made in the laboratory to treat cancer, rheumatoid arthritis, and other diseases.

Forms of biological therapy include interferon. The side effects of biological therapy depend on the type of treatment. Often, these treatments cause flu-like symptoms such as chills, fever, muscle aches, weakness, and loss of appetite, nausea, vomiting, and diarrhea. Some patients develop a rash, and some bleed or bruise easily. These side effects are usually short-term and they gradually go away after treatment stops.

Interferon beta-1a is sold under the trade name Rebif. An injection is used three times a week in the treatment of recurring multiple sclerosis.

I couldn't find any reference relating it to cancer treatment.

Papadakis explained that because Interferon hasn't been used on a child with cancer in Greece before, I would have to get any prescriptions from an IKA doctor. I made an appointment with yet another doctor at yet another hospital.

I outlined Lucy's story and the doctor, a solemn-faced middle-aged man in a black suit, dark grey shirt and tie, listened intently, asking for further details that Papadakis had given me from Lucy's file. He read quickly, turning the pages without comment.

'Your daughter must be a very strong little character. She's certainly gone through it all, hasn't she? I can support her doctor's proposal; I can verify the treatment and the prescriptions but you or your daughter will have to go before a committee to have it approved.' The doctor signed the paper and wished me all the best. It wasn't just a casual comment, he really meant it.

Then I started to worry. What if the committee didn't approve the Rebif interferon that Papadakis suggested? What if that meant changes in Lucy's medication? What if …? The thought has been in and out of my head for days.

Chris called to tell me that a car had hit her son, Henry. His leg was badly broken and he was hospitalised for several days. 'Several women at the hospital remarked on how calm I was,' she said. 'Well, were you?' I asked. 'Of course I wasn't. Inside I was falling apart, but I tried not to show it. I told the ladies about you and how you'd told me you weren't allowed to cry or show your fears in front of Lucy. How you continued to look on the bright side. And I did just the same!'

Is that really me?

How have I changed? How do I see and react to things? Am I softer or harder? Do others see the difference?

Monday 13 May

This morning I was again downtown in Athens to find another IKA office where the 'committee' (I saw only one woman but as she signed the paper and was very pleasant – I didn't question anything) approved the medication. I was directed to a specialised IKA pharmacy in an office building close to the bustling Omonia Square. For some reason I hadn't anticipated waiting and was shocked at the long queue of people patiently shuffling their way towards the service counter. I was probably the only healthy person there; most were obviously cancer patients and many didn't look well at all. It was heartbreaking.

The pharmacist checked my prescription, noted the committee's approval stamped on the reverse and asked, 'Who is the medication for?'

'My daughter.'

'How old is Loukia?'

'She's eight.'

'Do you have any identification with you, Mrs Mortzou?' I handed over my ID card, asking why it was necessary.

'Any medication that is available here is expensive and invariably strong. We must ensure there are no mistakes.' She smiled and continued. 'These injections must be kept in a refrigerator. Have you brought a freezer bag or anything similar with you?'

'No.'

'Where do you live?'

'Lucy and I live on Rhodes but we are staying at the Elpida hostel,' I explained.

'Okay, you must go straight back to the hostel. It's important that they are kept cool. Try and remember to bring an appropriate bag next time.'

I thanked her and left the building feeling like I was carrying a kilo of gold. I hailed a taxi and hurried straight back to the hostel. Lucy and I didn't have a fridge in our room so I stored them carefully in the fifth-floor refrigerator, removing one sealed injection to take with us to TAO.

I was dreading the first injection. The Interferon was one medication that couldn't be taken via her Hickman. Lucy was aghast when I explained that she would have one injection three times a week for six months.

'Oh, Mum.'

I tried to explain that I would help her through it.

'Yeah, great help you will be, as usual. You don't have to have the injection. You won't feel the pain.'

She was right of course. She wasn't, however, taking into consideration my pain in watching her suffer.

At TAO the ever-patient clinic sister explained that the injection should be taken at around the same time each day, carefully including

Lucy in any decision-making. 'Lucy, it's just before 10am. What do you say to making that the standard time for your Rebif? That way it is over and done with and you have your day free. Agreed?'

Lucy nodded reluctantly and watched as the sister coaxed her through the new medication. There was no immediate reaction, little pain (Lucy had winced but said it didn't really hurt, it was more of a burning sensation) and no noticeable side effects. Papadakis wanted Lucy to remain on the ward so he could watch her progress until the evening. She didn't mind, she had Alexandros and Antony for company and was, I thought, surprisingly lively and happy.

I ventured outside to chat with the other mothers on the TAO smoking terrace. Artemis was there, alone. We talked about Panayiota and then about little Elena and her battle over the past two years.

'Elena was just a normal, little two-and-half-year-old girl, running about everywhere, full of mischief, full of laughter, full of life,' she said, taking a long puff on her cigarette.

'She was quick, intelligent; fine until she caught what I thought was a cold. Her doctor said it was bronchitis and he prescribed a course of antibiotics.

'Elena didn't improve and started vomiting every morning. No one seemed to know what was wrong with her but her doctor suggested a stomach problem. He told me that she shouldn't be eating so much junk food. Can you imagine? Elena didn't eat junk food and told me herself that she didn't feel well. So we changed doctor and he talked about some pressure on the brain. Tests were made but nothing found.'

Artemis paused, took a sip of her coffee and continued. 'A month or so before Christmas, Elena started to notice smells, any smells, perfume, food, they all annoyed her. She also started to sleep a lot, much more than normal. I decided to try another doctor who wanted to treat Elena for worms. It was suggested that I had a problem, not my daughter.'

Artemis had stopped and sighed. Judy came into my thoughts. I recalled doctors telling my sister to take better care of her child when she had sought advice after Tania's initial convulsions. They told her to stop imagining things.

Artemis continued. 'I took her to a Christmas party, hoping that Father Christmas, the presents and the children would lift her spirits, but Elena slept. She just dozed heavily on my shoulder. By then she had started to stumble, wobble like a drunk, and it seemed her head was turning to one side all the time.

'I went back to the doctor and he suggested that Elena was dehydrated. Of course she was, by then she wasn't even drinking water. It was a nightmare! Or so I thought, never realising that the real nightmare was about to start.

'Elena was admitted to Rhodes Hospital and the director of the children's ward ordered scans and tests to be made early the next day. He was on his way home, walking out of the ward, when Elena convulsed and fell into a coma. Within hours I was told there was a problem, possibly a brain tumour. I was given three hours to return home and pack and then the doctor and aircraft were waiting at the airport.

'I was numb, didn't comprehend what was going on, probably didn't want to know what I was hearing. It was 1999, two days before Christmas and my little girl was undergoing major brain surgery. The surgeons were putting a valve in her head to relieve the pressure on her brain. Twenty-four hours later she had further surgery to remove the tumour. That was when we were told that the cancer had spread, already to her spinal cord and bone marrow. After all those weeks of wrong diagnoses everything happened so unbelievably quickly.

'After surgery Elena talked. She wanted her dummy and she wanted her comforter, a cuddly cover she has had since she was a baby. Wow, did she talk then. Talked and talked, but she never walked again. After five days on the neurological ward we moved to TAO, Elena had another operation to have a Hickman fitted and chemotherapy started.

'Three months passed and the chemo was stopped because Elena couldn't cope with it. Instead of saving her it was killing her, so she started what was classed as a lighter treatment. We returned to Rhodes for a few days but Elena was not the child I had left with.

'I was told she would live for six months. At one stage the TAO director had told me that I would never see my daughter run again. The other doctors kept me hopeful, kept me believing, but this one was so blunt. I hated him for it.

'You know how it is; you keep hoping for a miracle. My family and I turned to the church and ran from one to another hoping the miracle would happen.

'Back in Athens there were so many times when I felt I couldn't go on.

'But you do, don't you? You buy time, you dream on.

'Of course we were running back and forth to Athens every month for therapy, one day of treatment and she was always on antibiotics and other medicine to stop anything like an epileptic attack, which could be fatal.

'That's what happened; another convulsion brought us back here when you and I first met. We were at home in Rhodes and Elena took a fit. I knew what I had to do and got her straight into hospital. She seemed normal again but tests showed otherwise.

'And here we are.

'They've told me there is no return, there are no more therapies, there is no hope. But Elena will fight to the end. I know she will.'

We walked back into the clinic and I knew that conversation had changed our relationship. It had suddenly become more than a friendship. It was like Artemis was my sister.

Lucy stayed in TAO until the evening while her specialist checked for possible side effects, something like the flu, but he later sent us off. The beginning of her final treatment had seemed comparatively easy.

Tuesday 14 May

It's a wonderful early evening, there's a cloudless sky and out on our little balcony I could be anywhere except here! Lucy is downstairs in the playroom and I have been doing some work for my boss on the computer. It is one way of switching off from whatever is around me.

My mind is on news that awaited us on our return to Elpida yesterday.

On our first day here in Elpida Lucy and I had gone into the playroom to have a nose around and I got talking to an older couple and their little girl, Asiminna. Asiminna, dark with chubby cheeks and flashing eyes, had just completed her main treatment for leukemia and the family was looking forward to going home after spending many months in Athens.

Her father is a farmer, a rather heavy, gentle man, of few words. Apparently he'd been complaining of a backache, had gone to see his doctor, and after receiving results of some tests had been admitted to Agios Savas with a tumour on the spine.

I'm so sad and oh so mad at the same time. As if they haven't been through enough with their little girl! If there is a God what kind of God is he to have these hard-working, kind and considerate people go through all these traumas and heartache?

Lucy woke in the middle of the night with a high temperature, her first reaction to the treatment. I didn't panic. I called the clinic and they told me to watch the temperature closely. I gave her a mild painkiller and she slept after midnight. She was obviously unnerved by the change and how she felt. She was angry and unsure of herself but as soon as the temperature dropped she was fine again.

Thursday 23 May

Days, once again, have rolled by unnoticed. It's a bit like living in a daze here. Every Monday, Wednesday and Friday we go to the hospital for Lucy's injection. She doesn't want it. She cries, moans and pleads with the ever-patient nurses who don't want to upset her. They know that the thick liquid burns as it goes into her skinny little arm. They know they must do it, just as Lucy knows she must take it.

Lucy doesn't talk much about how she feels. Her appetite has improved and apart from a shadow on her face, the signs of the heavy radiotherapy have gone. It's when I see other little girls playing, their long hair blowing in the wind, falling all over the place, that I wonder how she feels. I feel a jealousy, a twinge that's hard to describe. I hate to admit that I resent their happiness and their freedom. It hurts. I feel like Lucy has been robbed of her innocence and I wonder if she will ever get over it.

Magda was rushed into hospital today with chronic stomach pains. Poor little thing, just add that to everything else! At the same time Antony, who has already had two bone marrow transplants, had a bad temperature and looked swollen and peaky. He was not his usual self and I felt sorry for him as he and his mother hurried off to TAO for tests.

They left Effy and I talking over coffee. We were numb, realising that as part of the Elpida family when one child is ill again all the parents cry and worry. Antony was somehow in front of me all night, behind my closed eyes as I struggled, unsuccessfully, to find the escape that sleep offered.

This delightful boy, polite and funny, with a great sense of humour and the ability to flirt with females of any age, declared one evening that he would marry Lucy. Well, Lucy was over the moon, she glowed with happiness while Antony had to placate an angry four-year-old Yorgos who was adamant that Lucy was his! Was I the only one left wondering if these children would grow up to marry?

On Sunday I called Mum for her birthday. She sounded good, happy and bright. 'My friends are still praying for Lucy here ... and they're working on getting you all over to this side of the world,' she chuckled.

I thanked her and them yet again, and suggested they add a few other names: Magda, Antony, Dimitri, Vaso and Elena to their prayer list.

Lucy has befriended little Asiminna, who was staying at the hostel with her mother while her father undergoes his first chemotherapy. She's a strange wee thing, extremely quiet, sucking and biting constantly on a rubber dummy. We babysat while her mother went to the hospital and each day this little character became more adventurous.

It was Lucy's idea to treat Asiminna to a ride in the battery-operated cars in St Thomas Square.

Bored and obviously dejected with the lack of business during the quiet late afternoon, the car operator was delighted to see us. He quickly charged cars for the girls and they were on their way, or rather Lucy was. Asiminna couldn't get the hang of the car at the beginning. She had it going backwards, then stalled to start again and head off crab-like in a sideways shuffle that would have been impossible to duplicate. Suddenly she took off and it was, quite simply, one of the funniest things I have ever seen. Asiminna had a ball; she laughed, sang and sparkled with delight. She also turned into a demon driver, a dab hand at ramming pedestrians' ankles, careering straight for the elderly ladies who dared to cross her path and whose afternoon stroll in St Thomas square would undoubtedly never be the same again. She drove like a bat out of hell until the little car started to slow and its battery finally died in front of the church steps. Both girls demanded another ride but I was aching from laughter. I bribed them away from the cars with ice creams, which sent Asiminna into another realm; she ate with a reverence for the taste of something new, something very special.

I happily relayed our outing to Asiminna's mother later that evening, when the poor woman quietly admitted that Asiminna had never been on a tricycle let alone in an electric car and that the ice cream was her daughter's first ever. Racked with guilt I apologised and felt awful until the next day, when I found mother and daughter in the same square sharing an ice cream after Asiminna's second car ride.

I have just turned a page here and found a red heart drawing.
'With love to my mum', it says.
Lucy often asks what I am writing, gets angry at times, but usually just leaves me to it. It's a special surprise because she rarely tells me that she loves me.

Elpida always goes out of its way to celebrate its young residents' birthdays and yesterday was no exception, with a combined party for Yorgos and another leukemia patient, two-year-old Eleni, a tiny fragile creature who has the makings of a great ballet dancer. Like a breakable doll, Eleni was known to roam the hostel either totally naked or dressed to the nines in frills and laces. Yesterday she was, predictably, in pink frills for the party, which wasn't held in the hostel's playroom. Elpida treated us all to a visit to the Attica Zoological Park, near Sparta.

The children's non-stop laughter and babbling started on the coach and continued as they were shown around the carefully landscaped private zoo, which had an impressive collection of birds. The animals shrieked and squawked along with their young visitors, who calmed down only when the tables were set with cakes and party favourites.

I noticed Josef had distanced himself from the other children. He was angry and unhappy.

'What's up Josef?'

'Go away! I don't want to talk to anyone. No one likes me here. No one wants to play with me.'

He was walking slowly, running his hands along the wire of the animals' cages, the noise making the little creatures scurry away in fright. 'Look, even the animals run away from me,' he cried, big tears streaking his sad little face.

'I bet if you touch the cage a little bit lighter, maybe even stop and wait a bit, the animals will come to you.'

'What do ya bet?' he scowled.

'Oh, I don't know. What can we bet? If I'm right then you have to come back and join the party. Okay?'

'Okay. But the rabbit won't come out,' he said falling on his knees in front of the cage. A few seconds passed without movement, and I feared I would lose the bet. But then the rabbit did venture out of its house and moved, like a magnet, to nuzzle into Josef's hand, his fingers locked around the cage wire. His face lit up in surprise and doubt. 'What should I do now?'

'Just stroke him through the wire,' I suggested. 'I think he wants to be your friend.'

'Wow! That's great. He's not running away. He likes me!'

'Of course he likes you … we all like you! Now you have to come back to the party 'cause I just won the bet.' Josef looked up, a small smile starting to spread across his face. He walked back to the party table and sat next to Lucy and another little Albanian boy. He was content, even more so when the zookeeper had him hold one of the colourful parrots.

'Well, would you look at that! This parrot – Billy is his name – doesn't usually like young visitors,' the zookeeper explained. 'Billy finds children a bit too noisy. He doesn't usually sit with anyone except me, but look now. He's certainly found a new friend in … what's your name?'

'Josef.'

'Well, Josef, you can come here any time and talk with Billy, because you've made him a very happy parrot.'

And Billy made Josef a very happy boy.

Saturday 25 May

Lucy's treatment continues without any major problems, apart from some dizziness and slight headaches. She loathes the injections but there is no alternative. (Probably just as well. If the Rebif was in liquid form Lucy could spit it out, as she so often does her antibiotics.) I have tried to tell her how much good it must be doing, but it's like talking to a wall.

Today we were out to meet my American friend Sheila, and her eight-year-old godchild, Kia, from Lindos. We met at a hamburger bar quite close to Agios Savas. They were in Athens to attend a performance of the San Francisco Ballet. I was reluctant to take Lucy because the closed theatre would be packed.

As the girls tucked into their lunches Sheila couldn't take her eyes off Lucy. 'What a difference since that last time I saw her. She's totally lost that gaunt look and her colour has changed. To be honest,' she said, 'she doesn't look anything like that little cancer child who was on Rhodes a couple of months ago. She looks great, which is more than I can say about you.' Sheila's standard diatribe on my weight and eating habits followed, but that was nothing new.

What was new, however, was that I had managed to change the Hickman fluid for the first time. I tried to explain the feeling to Sheila, but I think I lost her when I started describing shutting off the medication line.

It was something that I should have learned earlier but we'd always had the security blanket of the hospital being nearby and it seemed easier for the nurses to do it. Now we were getting ready to leave Athens I had to master it myself. At my first attempt in the TAO examination room I had Olivia, the patient nurse with the lovely smile and shining eyes, as my guide and I couldn't have wanted for a better teacher. She told Lucy to lie on the bed and asked me to control my shaking hands.

I took a deep breath. Right. I laid out the dressings, syringes, and new cap, sprayed to sterilise and managed to desterilise the gloves immediately. Another breath and back to the beginning.

Lucy, as always, lay dead still but her mouth never closed. She gave a flow of constant orders. 'Do this, do that, no not like that Mum,' until Olivia politely hushed her. I made sure the clip on Lucy's Hickman was open, syringed blood and fluid off and closed the clip. With the syringe full of the Heparin solution I reopened the clip, emptied the syringe, closed the clip, cleaned, put a new cap on and wiped again.

It wasn't easy. I was tense and worried about making a mistake, but Olivia said nothing, just nodded her head towards the end.

I will be totally on my own the next time. Who will be there to shut Lucy up then?

17

Tuesday 28 May

Today I woke feeling something was wrong. I didn't want to get out of bed.

Pia, my Swedish friend from Rhodes, called early and we had a coffee in the nearby square while Lucy was still in bed watching television. Pia needed documents from a nearby hospital before her husband could start radiotherapy in another clinic on the other side of the city. She too was in a difficult situation in Athens as she didn't have anyone to look after her children in Rhodes. Her elder daughter was studying for exams and the younger daughter and son were pretty wild. As we sat talking, Tula rushed by. She stopped when she saw me and left the key to her room at Elpida.

'Colleen can you do me a huge favour. I think I've left the iron plugged in. Can you check it for me?' Tula was stressed and shaking. She was in a terrible state.

I didn't have to ask what was wrong. She was running straight to intensive care and her precious niece.

I left Pia, wishing her and Manolis all the best, and returned to Elpida. Tula had left the iron on. It was lying on its side on top of the bed. I quickly turned it off and sat for a moment. At that time little Elena was fighting for what was left of her life.

I went to call Smaro to see if she and Dimitri would be out of the clinic today, but something stopped me. I didn't want to hear any bad news from Smaro. She had enough to worry about after Dimitri's bone marrow transplant. Strangely enough I left that call and found the courage to call Maria, Panayiota's mother.

Maria sounded good, strong but of course missing the teenager who had filled every minute of her life over the past two years. She asked after her 'little bud', her nice description for Lucy, who really was starting to blossom again. I wondered if Maria could regain her strength; refocus her life on her two children. Could she believe that Panayiota's fight was not all in vain?

I can't imagine being in her situation – or can I? It's a thought that's always at the back of my mind. It comes up and I quickly push it back, trying to concentrate on positive things, on things that are happening and not on the 'what ifs'.

At lunchtime, in the busy downstairs kitchen, I heard that Elena had died. Like Tania's death so long ago, we had been expecting the news for a long time, but when it came it hit really hard.

I was in the kitchen with Nico's mother, Maria, when Magda's mum Yorgia came in from TAO. We were busy cooking and talking. Yorgia stopped to lean on the doorframe. She was uncharacteristically quiet. I looked up and saw that she'd been crying. She met my gaze and the tears started.

'She's gone. Elena's gone.'

I opened my mouth to speak but had no words. I needed air and turned slightly to pass through the door on to the balcony. Yorgia joined me, offering me a cigarette. No one spoke, no one moved; we just sobbed silently, the only sound coming from our deep drags on the cigarettes.

Elena had gone and we were lost. She'd been fighting for so long, battling against an enemy that, no matter what, would not give up. The doctors had tried everything, but it just wasn't enough. Elena didn't stand a chance.

Elena's few words to Lucy had included 'I love you'. The girls had related in a way that I couldn't understand, little minds and souls touching, knowing each other and feeling each other's hurt and pain.

Today I feel I have lost a daughter, a very precious little girl, who didn't have a chance. Artemis and Tula were strong and smiling until the end. I want to hug them, take some of their pain away, but they've gone already.

Yorgia told us that another Elpida child, little Eleni, who also stayed on the fifth floor, had been rushed in to intensive care with breathing difficulties. I had gotten to know Eleni's shy parents a few weeks prior to their departure for specialised radiotherapy in a London clinic, before going into the Agia Sofia transplant unit. They were worried about the trip and I had asked Chris to go and see them. She'd taken toys for Eleni and arranged for a Greek-speaking nurses' aide to help them. They had been so grateful when they returned to the hostel. They had told me their plans for when their little Eleni was well again.

What plans would that poor couple be making now?
Enough God. Can you hear me? It's more than they can take.
Don't push and hurt these children and their parents any more.

Amidst all that pain, Smaro and Dimitri are out of the unit. He's fragile, even smaller than before, a little bird with huge brown eyes. I can't see that wonderful flash of a smile as he's wearing a mask all the time.

Dimitri is unsure, wary. He looks ready to break he is so small. I want to take him in my arms and somehow bring back the joy that he had before going into the unit, the laughter trying to find a taxi, a silly bottoms knocking game he and I had played in the hostel corridor. He's like a wounded little bird who is scared to try his wings again.

Smaro is happy to be out of the transplant unit but full of doubts of how to cook for her son, how to care for him in a normal environment. Normal! The hostel isn't normal, it's not real life and now that I know Lucy and I will soon be returning to real life and our home, I feel it even more.

The security here is something I have never really felt during all my years in Greece. It's something that my husband, despite the love we shared for many years, never gave me. I have found security through Lucy's illness, in a hostel for children with cancer.

Does anyone else share my feelings, a reluctance to leave after all these months of missing our former life?

I have written an article for the hostel newsletter. It took a long time. No, that's not quite true. It's written from the heart and didn't take me long; it just took time to get it right. Maybe this article explains how I feel.

I will never forget the day I was told that Lucy was ill.

It was just a normal Saturday morning I guess … warm for that time of year (early December), the festive season was getting into swing and I was sitting watching my little girl. She'd had surgery on her neck the day before, was still groggy but obviously happy that it was all over.

One of the many doctors we had seen over the past two days was at the door. 'Mrs Mortzou, could you come into my office for a moment please?'

I felt weighed down by some kind of darkness, dread. I shrugged it off as tiredness, until the doctor started talking. She was telling me that Lucy had a problem and that chemotherapy had to start as soon as possible. I couldn't take it in – didn't want to take it in. The whole thing didn't fit into my already tired and numb brain.

I stumbled out of the doctor's office and collided with a couple laughing in the corridor. Laughing! I wanted to spit at them and hit them. How dare they laugh and act as if everything was normal?

My life, Lucy's very young life, had just been shattered, blown apart. I felt an arm around my shoulder and another doctor told me to relax, I mustn't show any signs of anguish or worry, I mustn't cry in front of Lucy.

'You have a long road ahead of you, you must be strong for your little girl and for yourself,' she said.

Strong? I was walking but couldn't feel my legs, talking without making sense. Thank goodness Lucy was groggy from the previous day's surgery. She has always been quick to read my thoughts and reactions but that day she didn't remark on my stumbling speech and raw, red eyes. She just slept and mumbled, she didn't complain at all, and I stared at the soulless hospital walls hoping, praying, I would wake from this ghastly nightmare and find everything back to normal.

I didn't wake of course.

The nightmare just got worse as Lucy's illness became reality and our lives were changed forever. I visited the TAO clinic and the panic that was clawing my stomach increased. No, I could never take my Lucy there. The children had no hair, they were wired to all sorts of medicines; she would freak out, I thought.

Lucy, however, did move into TAO a few days later. I had worried myself sick that she would withdraw into herself, shy away from any company. She didn't. She took one look at the surroundings, the children in the ward and minutes later she was swapping stickers, sketching and colouring with the other children. For goodness sake, she was laughing!

Six months have passed since those first few days. Six months of treatment, hospitals, doctors, and medicines. Six months of good days and bad days, of laughter and tears, of making new friends and losing precious faces.

Half a year of a new life ... no, the same life seen through different eyes.

Want it or not, Lucy and I have become part of another family, an unusual family where there are no relations, no blood ties. It's a family in which the bonding, however, is so strong, the friendship, the smiles – and sometimes tears – so real that I almost believe that her illness was part of a plan to make us better people, to open our eyes, our hearts to something that we had taken for granted before.

Life.

Through the hours spent in TAO, the months at Elpida, I have discovered that I wasn't living. Sure I was alive, fighting to look after my children, working, always on the run, on the edge, with little or no time to appreciate the simple things in life – a smile, children's laughter, their singing and dancing, the understanding in the eyes of someone who has become more than a friend.

I thought Lucy's illness was the end of my world but it was just another beginning ...

Lucy's specialist found me in the TAO waiting room last evening. Lucy had gone to TAO to see the girls from the Children's Smile Group. Funny, she bounded in there as if she was at home and didn't want to leave when it was time to return to the hostel.

Papadakis chatted about Athens, its museums, Microlimano and sailing as a child, his own family.

'We've fixed a date, 7 June, for Lucy's next CT scan. This will be the big one at this stage. It will show what we have achieved and if …' Papadakis left the sentence unfinished. 'No ifs,' he added. 'I'm sure Lucy can continue her treatment on Rhodes so you should be thinking about heading home again.' He smiled and hurried towards his office. He did not mention a date for heading home.

Later I changed the fluid in Lucy's Hickman by myself, without a trusty nurse hovering nearby. Lucy wasn't the ideal patient ('do this, do that'), I had an awful fluttering in my stomach and, of course, my hands shook, but I managed.

Sunday 2 June

Routine is probably the best description for the past few days. Lucy has been into TAO for her injections and to check on her friends in the clinic (great news: little Marina, who was with us at the beginning of Lucy's treatments, had her Hickman taken out today, and her normally sombre parents were beaming) and we have been making the most of balmy summer days with other friends from the hostel.

With Maria and Nico we set out to sample some of Athens' history, starting with the Greek Parliament Building in Syntagma Square. We arrived just in time for the changing of the guards outside this former palace, so Lucy and Nicos watched intently as the striking young Evzones marched and paraded. The Evzone fighters go a long way back in Greece's history and remain an important icon. It was their uniform, the 'foustanella' cotton skirt, which captured the children's attention. We moved on to wander the National Gardens, which, I hated to admit, I had never really noticed. It was a fresh, cool change from the bustle of downtown Athens and the park was surprisingly well kept and clean. We walked on to the impressive Zappeion Exhibition Hall and crossed the busy street leading towards the one and only Panathenaiko or Kalimarmaro Stadium of the 1896 Olympic Games.

—

Two days later the children decided on another tour through central Athens, but this time they were not interested in walking. Lucy and Nicos had seen a bright little tourist train during our wander and demanded we try it. Yorgia's Magda was not going to be left out.

Once there, our Elpida children laughed, sang, greeted anyone and everyone. They were three happy-go-lucky children without any cares in the world.

—

This evening the hostel was invited to the local school's end-of-year party. Elpida children were given the best seats to watch the school children perform traditional Greek songs and dances. It was a bright, lively atmosphere. During the school's awards ceremony its basketball team was presented with a cup they had won in a local competition. Lining up to be congratulated by the school's principal, the young athletes turned to the seated Elpida children and one of the boys took the microphone.

'We'd like you to have this award', he said, his gaze taking in all the children. 'This is in recognition of the game that you guys are playing and the fact that you are all winners.'

The Elpida parents, including myself, were flabbergasted. What a nice thought, what a great way of saying, 'Hey, we know you can't play any sports at the moment, but we also know why. Just keep fighting and you'll get there just like we did!'

Dimitri was sitting behind Lucy and Josef. He leaned forward and tapped them on their shoulders. 'Go on you two. You go and accept that cup on behalf of all your friends at Elpida.'

Lucy and I returned to Elpida brighter, somehow lighter, than a few hours earlier.

18

Monday 3 June

Good feelings, it seems, aren't meant to last long.

Lucy woke this morning complaining of sore legs and a headache.

'It's probably from all the excitement last night,' I told her, treating her complaints lightly until she returned to our room from the small bathroom. She was crying, with big tears sliding silently from wide, frightened eyes.

'I think I have a lump again, Mum,' she said, moving her right hand to the side of her neck.

I tried desperately not to show the panic that filled my mouth, my lungs, and my stomach.

'Here, let me see. Luce, there's nothing there,' I said, lightly rubbing the side of her tiny neck, and then wiping away her tears. 'You're probably just tired. There's no reason to cry. Come on, let's see if Yorgia and Magda are still here and we'll go to TAO with them this morning. Go and knock on their door.'

For once she did exactly as she was told. I didn't have to tell her that I had felt something, that her neck did seem to be swollen.

Shit! My hands were shaking; my heart was pounding so hard it seemed to be beating through my ears. A quick glance in the mirror told me I would have to hide the look I saw. I couldn't let Lucy know my fears. I took a deep breath, closed our door and turned to see Lucy and Magda walking arm-in-arm towards the lift.

The little imp turned back to look at me. 'We're going in the mini bus today,' she said. 'Can Lucy come with us? Say yes, please, please, say yes!'

Yorgia and I looked at one another, smiled, and I nodded agreement. The girls laughed together in the lift. For the moment, Lucy had forgotten her neck. Yorgia, however, was quick to read my face. 'What's up? What's wrong? You two were so happy and pretty last night. What's happened? Has Lucy been off with you again?'

'I wish,' I said, and quickly explained what had happened. Yorgia squeezed my arm, told me not to worry and thought I didn't see the slow, long breath she had taken.

In TAO Lucy surprised the nurses by putting up no resistance to her injection. She was quiet and they and her specialist understood that something was wrong.

'Okay, Lucy. Let's see what's happening here,' he said as he held her neck between his hands. His mouth twisted slightly when he found something he didn't like, but to Lucy he said, 'It's probably the start of a cold or maybe your radiation treatment still doing some work there. I want you to stay here though until lunchtime so that I can keep an eye on you.

'I'm pretty sure it's nothing to worry about,' he said.

Easier said than done I'm afraid.

After a rather difficult few hours in TAO Lucy returned to the hostel miserable and, I thought, tired. I sat on the side of our bed and thought about reading for a while and Lucy was suddenly in front of me, hands on her hips. She was angry.

'I want a Playstation. All the other kids have a Playstation. I want one. You never get me what I want.'

She started to scream, lunging out and trying to hit and scratch me. It was awful. Her tantrum was a long one. It left her voiceless and with an even more swollen neck. She was wild and I couldn't stop her. I felt helpless and incredibly alone. As a last resort I called Dimitri and his assistant, Nicoletta, for help.

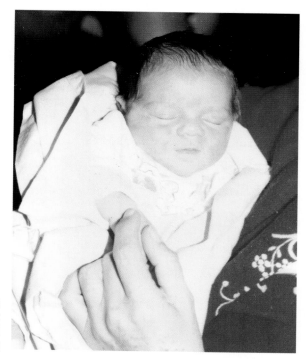

Loukia May Mortzou, born Thursday 17 February 1994 at 8.50am in the Rhodes General Hospital; weight 3.45 kg

"One of the boys" – a typically mischievous Lucy, always ready to beat her brothers at the popular game of tapas

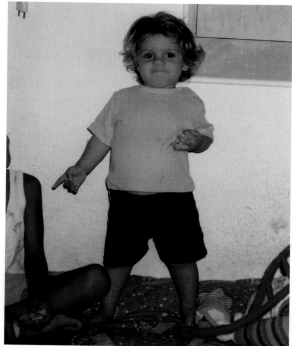

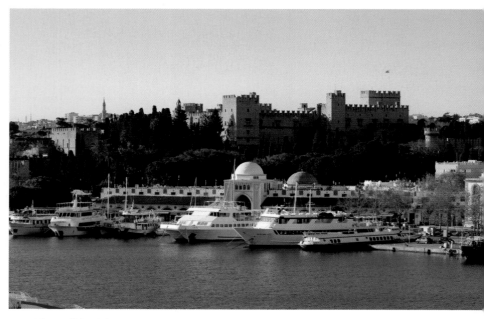

The striking Mandraki Harbour area in Rhodes city centre, with the medieval Palace of the Grand Master of the Knights of Rhodes that dominates the walled Old Town

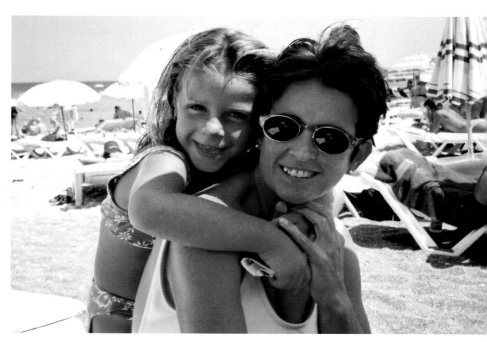

Lucy and me at Elli Beach some months before we flew to Athens

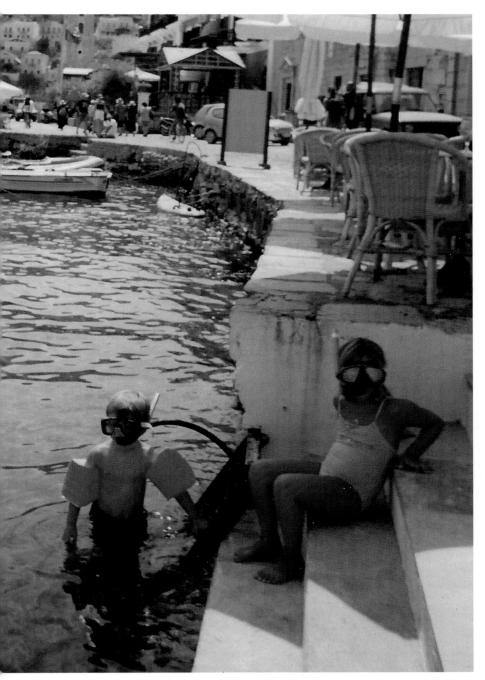

On Symi: Lucy coaxed the younger Henry into the crystal-clear water, teasing him into more daring swimming and diving

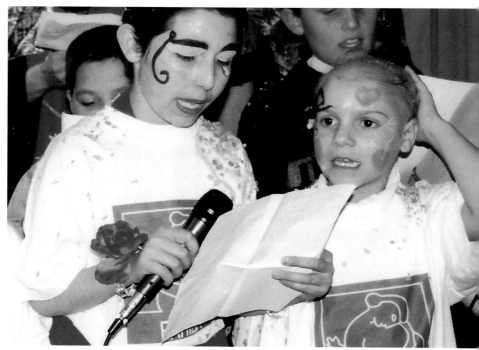

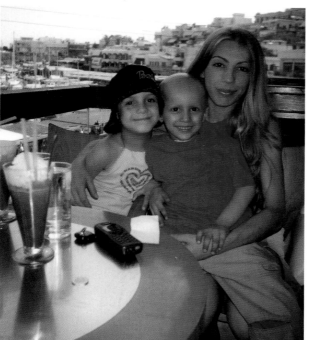

Above

Lucy with Maria Bousia, one of her many hostel friends, wearing t-shirts with the Elpid emblem during the Mardi Gras party at Elpida hostel

Left

Escaping from the daily routin of hostel, hospital and tests, Lucy out with Effy and her sor Yorgos (also from Rhodes) for iced coffee and chocolate near Microlimano (Small Port), a short drive from Athens

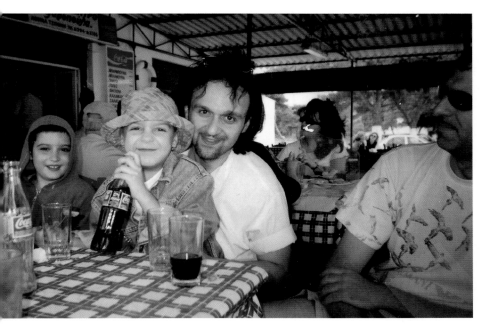

Lucy with Dimitri, her much-loved Elpida social worker,
and Katerina, another Elpida and TAO friend

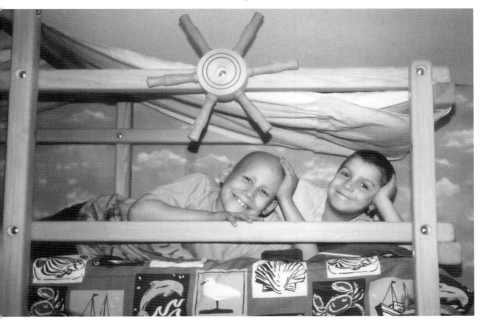

Alexandros and Lucy – a very special relationship with a very special little boy,
here on his new bunk bed courtesy of Make A Wish

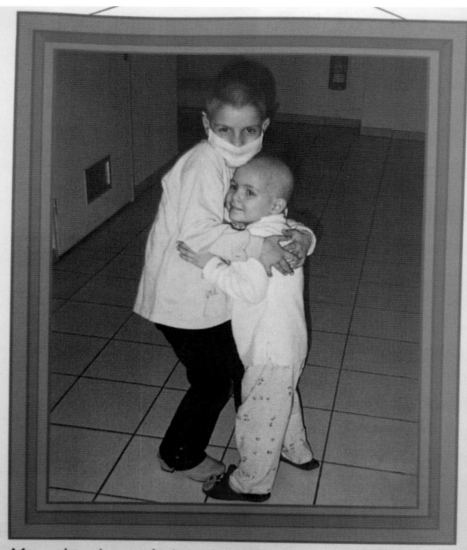

Μια σφιχτή αγκαλιά από την Λουκία στην Μάγδα είναι η καλύτερη ευχή για να μπει στη Μονάδα Μεταμόσχευσης Μυελού των Οστών.

Καλή επιτυχία, Μάγδα

Lucy and Magda as featured in the Elpida newsletter. The caption reads: 'A big hug from Lucy shows her best wish to Magda before she enters the bone marrow unit'

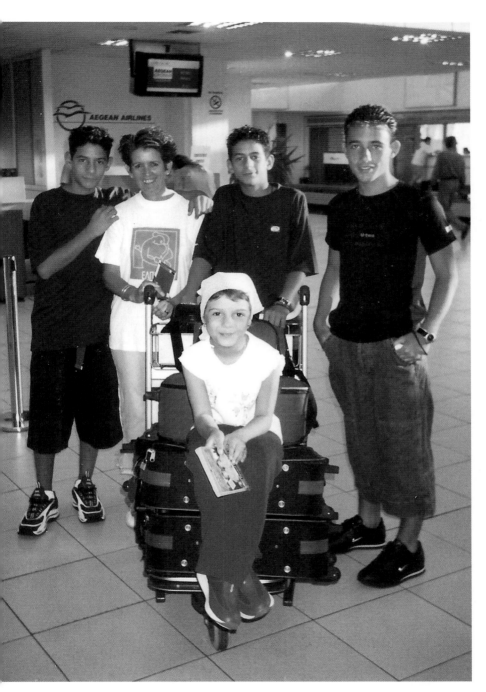

At Rhodes Diagoras Airport at the start of Lucy's
Make A Wish adventure: Sam (left), Tony and Yanni

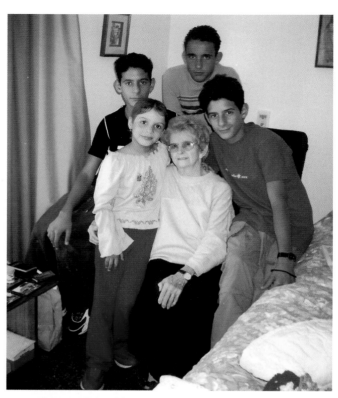

Left

Lucy's wish came true, with her Nana May Theresa Morgan and her brothers

Below

Lucy with her Nana, in a photograph that appeared in the *Press* newspaper, Christchurch (Fairfax Media/The *Press*)

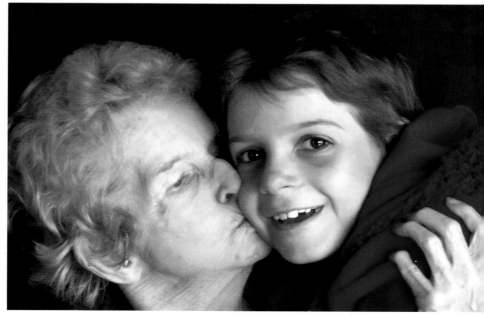

Dimitri spoke to Lucy and agreed to lend her a Playstation only if she stopped being so difficult.

God, clear my brain please. It's 2am and I have been trying to sleep for more than two hours.

Could Lucy be sick again? Could that swelling be a sign that the cancer has returned? Normally I can change my thoughts if that dark dread creeps back into my head, but not tonight. Tonight it seems that death is dancing around me. It's a horrible, hopeless feeling that won't go away.

Lucy is asleep beside me. To switch on the light I had to uncurl her fingers from my arm. She is scared and uncertain as well.

God, Lucy is eight years old, she shouldn't be experiencing all this.

Panayiota, Vasilis, Pandelis and Elena are in front of me.

Four young children who died suffering. God, that's a horrible word.

Lucy has had a bad day and I, as usual, have had a bad day with her. She's been sore, angry, aggressive, and abusive. But I wonder. How does she feel, what does she think when she sees girls her own age laughing, playing, jumping, without any cares? God, it's so sad, so wrong.

Lucy's asleep now, angel like with her hand on the pillow cupping her face. She's breathing easy. If she was ill again, it would show now, wouldn't it?

Little Dimitri is back in the transplant unit, that's bothering me as well. He had a temperature last night and he was quickly readmitted to Agia Sofia. Haven't he and his lovely mother been through enough?

Thursday 6 June

Thursday afternoon. I have been running, walking, all morning to arrange for two months' supply of Rebif injections. Without intending to, I managed to walk from the hospital to Omonia Square, the commercial hub of modern downtown Athens. It was a long walk but I needed it. Somewhere along the busy bustling streets I managed to clear my head.

I'm not feeling well. It's as if my mind and body are focused on Lucy's scan tomorrow. So much depends on that test. It will prove the doctors right or wrong; it will show what, if anything, remains of the tumour and if there are any other problems. It is the key to Lucy's future and to mine.

It's as if there is a noose around my neck and someone is slowly but surely choking me. I can't concentrate – even writing this, an attempt to put words to my thoughts and feelings, is a struggle.

Lucy's difficult, not wanting to shower, shouting, angrier than she has been for some time. Is this return to aggression a result of the Interferon? I watch and wait for reactions. Her neck seems swollen one minute and fine the next. I am searching for symptoms.

She's not eating and is nervous and edgy. The only time she smiles is when she's with Dimitri who has returned to Elpida, smaller and more delicate than before. Lucy loves that little boy and appears to forget her own problems when she is with him. Unfortunately that's not very long as the poor child still has a temperature so neither he nor Smaro can relax.

Friday 7 June

Lucy and I were up early and into TAO before the everyday rush of outpatients. We weren't in the TAO waiting room more than five minutes before the clinic's secretary filled my arms with Lucy's folder and directed us downstairs to the CAT scan and x-ray area.

After about 40 minutes' waiting a nurse approached us and said, 'Lucy it's your turn now. Do you want your mother in there as well?'

'No, I'm okay this time,' Lucy smiled. She moved into the scan room alone. She knew the routine and was no longer daunted by the huge machine, the noise, the periods of silence and the waiting.

Sitting outside I was the opposite of Lucy's calmness. I felt as if we had been taken back to the beginning again, the only difference being that Lucy knew exactly what was expected of her.

I felt numb and nauseous. The scan took longer than usual and Lucy was tired when we returned to TAO to be told that the results wouldn't be known until Monday.

Mina, the quietly spoken sympathetic doctor on the TAO team, read my fears. She smiled and shrugged slightly before moving off towards the doctors' office. I was ready to burst into tears, but I didn't, I did what most of the anguished, waiting parents always did. I sighed, took a deep breath and tried to bury my feelings.

I had work to do and Lucy said she'd help. The hostel was planning a picnic over the weekend and all the mothers were making something so we left the hospital, shopped at the supermarket and headed straight into the Elpida kitchen to prepare a typical New Zealand picnic dish, a bacon and egg pie. I was happy to have something to do as I didn't want time to think what the scan could show.

Concentrating on the pie, I felt a hand on my arm. It was Katerina's mother, Eleni.

'Colleen, where have you put your cell phone? Mina has been trying to contact you for ages.'

My whole body started to shake and I could feel (hear?) my pounding heart as I moved to find my phone in my bag. The two eggs in my hands splattered on the kitchen floor; the paper bag with the remaining flour spilled, spreading like a cloud over the bench space. It took just a moment but I felt time had stopped.

Eleni touched my shoulder. 'Wait. Calm down,' she said. 'There's no reason to call now. Mina said the scan was fine.'

Relief flooded through my body, tears streaming down my cheeks as I looked at Eleni's smiling face. I kissed her. I wanted to hug everyone. God I felt good. I wanted to call the hospital but by the time I found my phone at the bottom of my bag I was calmer and listened to my friends.

'There's no reason to call now,' Eleni said. 'You know that it's good, we don't need the details. Let's not bother them at TAO; they've got enough on their plate!'

I celebrated with a strong coffee and called Lucy to get ready for our evening visit to Alexandros.

He didn't know that we'd be visiting. We'd been invited to his home for a Make a Wish surprise. Alexandros' wish was for a new bedroom. Make A Wish had excelled, turning a drab child's bedroom into a cabin fit for an outgoing, adventure-loving captain, Captain Alexandros. His face was a picture when he arrived home to find the living room filled with TAO mothers.

Easygoing Alexandros shrugged his shoulders, lifted his eyebrows slightly and moved to open the door to his room. He wasn't aware of the many eyes watching his movements and he strode into the room without – for a second or two – registering anything unusual. Then he turned to look at his mother, his eyes full of wonder. His 'Mum!' hadn't left his mouth before a chorus of his younger guests sprang up from their hiding places beneath the chunky duvets covering his brand new wooden bunk beds.

'Surprise!' they shouted, and clambered off the beds to greet their friend, who was slowly taking in the changes to his room. 'I got my wish,' he said over and over again. 'Wow!' He was one very happy little boy. The delight, the wonder and the happiness on his face will be etched in my mind forever.

Lucy was quick to tire. She'd had a big day and didn't want to party, so we returned to the hostel to be greeted by an ecstatic Pagona. I had just turned the key to unlock our door.

'Close it again, Colleen,' she said, hugging Lucy close to her side and leading her to a seat next to Antony. 'Come and have a drink with us. We've got some good news, haven't we Tony?' Her son smiled into Lucy's eyes and then met mine. A wide smile, his eyes suddenly brimming with tears. He said, 'I'm going home. I've finished with TAO and Elpida. We've packed up the room and we're going back to Zakynthos. We're going to be a family again.'

I looked from Tony to Pagona, to Christos and then to Lucy and realised we were all crying.

It was a bittersweet farewell. It was great that Antony was leaving but sad not knowing when we would see them again. I'm still sipping at the whisky Pagona topped up before we headed to our room after long hugs and a touching parting between Antony and Lucy.

Cheers, Antony. Here's to a future without sickness and problems. I promise that Lucy and I will dance at your wedding.

Tuesday 11 June

It's Tuesday evening and we are packed, ready to return to Rhodes.

How long have I been waiting to say that? To leave Athens? Lucy has the all clear from her specialist to return home, and I am sitting here questioning everything.

Yesterday we were into TAO on the hostel shuttle bus early, which has become a bit of a habit. Not a bad one, as usually there was no rush to get into the clinic for Lucy's injection. She chatted to her friends and I waited to speak to Papadakis. He hadn't seen me waiting and I managed to catch his eye as he made the morning round of the clinic with the team of doctors.

'As soon as we are finished I will call you', he said and he did.

'I can hardly believe what we are seeing here,' he said with a big smile on his face. 'The results are even better than we had expected. There are some spots, small marks, still showing on the scan but I'm pretty sure they will also disappear. Lucy's looking good, so good in fact that we can do without seeing you for a while.'

He was watching for my reaction and obviously saw the relief on my face. He smiled. 'We've done well haven't we? Lucy's done well, she's a remarkable child. She'll need to be careful, but I believe Lucy will be fine.'

Pausing a moment he spotted Lucy and called her over. 'Little Miss Rhodes, can you tear yourself away from your good-looking admirers for a moment and give me a minute of your time?'

Lucy grinned.

'You know what, Lucy? I'm tired of seeing you here nearly every day.'

Lucy looked uncertain and looked at me questioningly, as if she had done something wrong.

'I think it is time for you to get out of here and go home to your brothers!'

Lucy looked at him, looked at me, hugged her specialist and hurried off to share her good news with her friends.

I must have appeared very calm and collected to all around me but I wasn't at all; I couldn't really accept that it could be nearly over.

I noticed a distant, subdued and quiet Joanna by the clinic door. I caught her eye and a tear rolled slowly down her face as we headed out the door together to the smoking room. Alexandros and Lucy were chatting and laughing, arms around each other, heads close together, two little souls enjoying each other's company.

Joanna couldn't talk at first, her hand shaking as she tried to light a cigarette. She gulped down the smoke and said nothing.

'What is it?'

She shook her head and drew heavily on the cigarette. 'It's back,' she said, 'and this time it looks like it is here to stay.'

I couldn't believe my ears, didn't want to believe. Alexandros had always been so full of life, so bright, the sunshine and smile of the clinic, especially for Lucy on her many down days.

I had been ready to celebrate, and Joanna was fighting to accept the news that her little boy was dying.

Struggling to hide my feelings, I returned to the clinic, prised a beaming Lucy away from company and headed to the hostel. A phone call from TAO, however, sent us off in the opposite direction. We had to show the scan to Agios Savas. Fortunately even that long walk couldn't curtail Lucy's happiness. She led the way and bounded through the hospital to find her specialists.

Zampaties crouched down to hug Lucy.

'That's my girl, that's what we needed to see!' He looked at Thanos and both men beamed with relief.

'One day you'll realise just how happy you've made us Lucy,' Thanos said as he tousled Lucy's short hair. 'We've missed you, but, you know what? I hope we never see you again.'

'You won't,' said Lucy. 'I'm not coming back here. I'm going home.'

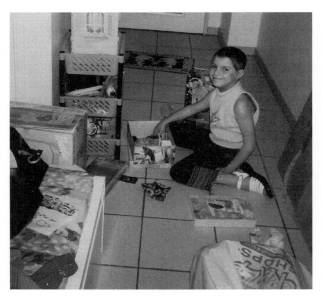

Lucy in our hostel room not long before our departure, happy and confident, about packing up her toys for Rhodes

We left Agios Savas full of best wishes from everyone there, even those patients we didn't know. They'd quickly realised that Lucy was the little girl they'd heard about, the little hero that had brightened the radiotherapy department.

I was exhausted but I decided to write another article for the hostel's magazine.

Yesterday was an important day.

It was a Monday just like any other Monday, but a very special one for Lucy and me. Her doctor saw us sitting in the TAO waiting room and asked what we were doing there! Why we weren't in Rhodes?

When he saw our puzzled expressions he explained that within the next two weeks, after a CAT scan, we could go home and continue some treatment there.

We had been waiting for weeks to hear those words and yet when we left the hospital half an hour later to return to Elpida, I started to wonder what they really meant.

Great, they meant that Lucy was getting better, that the worst of her treatment was over, the door back to our normal life was being reopened. Wonderful news, yet a funny feeling had taken over. There was a weight in my stomach and somewhere in my throat, a worry and a feeling that we would be leaving so much behind us in Athens.

I thought about the day we moved in to Elpida. Lucy definitely did not want to stay; she said she didn't like the look of the place.

She and I saw Elpida like a hotel at first. It didn't take long for us both to realise though, that Elpida is something much more, something very special.

Through Lucy's eyes it was first just a building. Quickly, she and I learnt more about the amazing people who, fortunately, are able to give not just their money, but also their time, to make and keep the building going.

At the same time we became attached to those within the hostel, fantastic people who don't just work there; it isn't as simple as that! Individually they are all experts in their own fields; they are also very special people. A smile, a word of advice, a touch on your shoulder, or a look that tells you they know and understand what you are going through. As a team they have produced that Elpida feeling that is so difficult to put into words, a feeling that grows and strengthens the longer you are there.

It's a feeling that enables you to put aside your worries and problems, it makes you realise that even on your worst days there is something to smile or laugh about.

Even now I don't think about the medicines, the heavy radiation treatment, the difficult days and sleepless nights that have become part of our lives. Elpida memories include being a blushing blue-faced bride again (now that was an experience I hadn't planned on, especially when my 'groom' was one of my wonderful new friends! Guess I should explain that we were married during a Mardi Gras party), and experiencing all the children performing at the same party (then the carefully applied light blue makeup and flowers ran together. I explained to Lucy that the tears were, as always, brought on by an allergy. Somehow she didn't believe me!). My head is full of the evenings spent around the tables in the dining room, sharing wonderful meals with new friends, watching the children laughing and playing together like old mates; peeking in on the kids' art therapy, their dancing and music lessons (am I the only one who feels a touch of magic in the air then?), fighting back the tears of astonishment at the children's theatre we shared, marvelling at the children's sparkling eyes during a trip to the Sparta Zoo. Tear-jerking birthday and farewell parties were full of surprises and laughter. All special moments touched by that magical Elpida wand – like the wand held by a wonderful good fairy intent on wiping out the darkness and doubt of our real world – that has watched over us during our stay in Athens.

Lucy's doctor has said we can go. Yes. It is going to be great returning home but it is also going to be difficult leaving this secure little haven. Perhaps the best part of it all is knowing that Elpida's door never closes ...

P.S. Thanks a million to all who are part of Elpida and to the wonderful friends and children who have, in a difficult time, enriched my life.

Later in the afternoon the children were treated to a surprise visit by a well-known Greek singer, Notis Sfakinakis. He was unassuming, signed CDs for the children and gave them all t-shirts. He came to visit Angelos, an 11-year-old from Corfu, who was a newcomer to the hostel. Angelos and his family had rocked the hostel on their arrival. They were noisy and Angelos was abusive and foul mouthed. He didn't want to be in Elpida, he didn't want to be with his parents and grandmother and he let everyone know with his loud tirades, which started early in the morning and continued until late at night.

Shocked initially, we quickly realised that Angelos' short temper and bad manners were a result of operations and therapy. He'd calmed down and was a nice kid with a wonderful smile when and if he wanted to be. Angelos had a large valve in part of his brain and didn't really look great. I suspected he didn't have long to live.

This special day had no end, it seemed. As we walked back from the singer in the Elpida lounge, Chris, one of my oldest friends from New Zealand, called to say she was staying in central Athens with friends who couldn't wait to see us. I thought Lucy would quickly decline her offer of dinner in a Plaka restaurant, but I was wrong. There was no stopping her today. We took a taxi downtown to meet Chris and her friends wandering through the fascinating streets and shops of the Plaka district. Exhausted from bartering with the shrewd Athenian shopkeepers, the Australasian tourists suggested dinner and we settled for a corner table in a taverna with spotless blue and white gingham tablecloths, fresh flowers and a great atmosphere. It was an evening full of smiles, laughter and stories. Lucy and my Peter Pan friend bonded quickly. There was no age barrier to their immediate friendship or the watermelon-pip spitting war they had, which could only be welcomed and encouraged in a friendly Greek tavern.

The competition, which left Lucy red-faced with laughter and disbelief that my close friend could prompt such outrageous behaviour, will no doubt be continued on Rhodes as Chris and her friends fly out of Athens tomorrow morning.

We will see them at home ...

Friday 21 June

We are home. We've been back on Rhodes for ten days and every day I have meant to open this journal ... the thoughts remain but I've put nothing to paper.

The days pass in a blur.

Lucy is my first and last thought, a constant worry. Now there are so many other things to do as well. Over the past months I have yearned to have my normal life back – now I wonder if that has gone forever.

I am tired. I look tired and feel tired. I'm up at the crack of dawn to clean and get this small house feeling like home again. It was dirty, dusty, full of cobwebs and not at all good for Lucy. It's clean now but I know that we must move from this old place that can be so cold, draughty and damp during the winter months.

On the evening we left Elpida I shut our main suitcase and sat on the end of my bed. I should have been elated but instead I felt rather lost, empty. I had hoped to spend the evening with Maria, Smaro and Effy, but that seemed impossible. Maria told me she was going to her sister's, Smaro had to visit her aunt and Effy had arranged to see a friend. I felt really disappointed but tried not to show it. I decided to write. I couldn't even do that. The hostel seemed deadly quiet, matching my mood of feeling lost and lonely. I had looked forward to a final evening with my new friends.

Dimitri appeared at the door.

'Ah, Colleen, I thought I might find you here. Any chance of you and Lucy coming down to the playroom for a moment? We have a newcomer to the hostel today and I'd like you to help welcome him.'

That's odd. Since when did Elpida welcome newcomers? If Dimitri saw the questioning look on my face, he didn't show it. 'Sure, why not?' I called Lucy and we headed towards the lift to go down to the basement playroom.

'Hang on a second,' Effy shouted. 'Yorgos and I will come down as well.'

The lift door opened at the basement level. Surprisingly, the door into the hall leading to the laundry and onto the playroom was closed. It was unusually quiet. I looked back at Effy but her face was showing no surprise, she just pointed for me to open the door. I did. The short corridor was empty and all the doors off the corridor were closed.

'I don't think there is anyone down here,' I said. 'In all the months we've been here, I've never seen all the doors closed. Where on earth is Dimitri?'

Effy shrugged and rather impatiently urged me to open the door leading to the playroom. I gingerly turned the handle and the door opened – onto a playroom full of our friends! A beaming Maria, Smaro and Yorgia, their children and other faces and friends from Elpida. They moved aside as we went into the room. There was a huge banner that read, 'We will Miss You, We Love You,' and a two-tier cake with a ceramic statue of the Colossus of Rhodes in the middle of it.

I laughed and I cried. I really didn't know what to do. I was overwhelmed and Lucy was basking in the limelight of a surprise farewell party, complete with a clown and many, many presents.

Hugs, kisses, smiles and tears. I tried to express my gratitude to Dimitri. 'Don't thank me,' he said. 'You have to thank your friends who know just how much they will miss you and Lucy.'

It was something special, very special, realising that these friends would miss us as much as we would miss them. I was lost for words – still am –

thinking of their love and thoughts. I too will miss them, their love, their friendship and their support. I know I will miss the security of Elpida as Lucy and I venture back to our real world, a world that part of me doesn't really want to return to.

How ridiculous is that? After all Lucy and I have been through I don't want to return to reality. I don't want to, or I am scared to?

I find myself watching Lucy, looking at her and wondering if the worst is over. I'm also secretly dreading whatever awaits us on Rhodes.

My feelings weren't unfounded. As soon at the plane's wheels touched the tarmac of Diagoras Airport on Rhodes, Lucy was trying to unbuckle her seatbelt. There was no holding her back and passengers moved out of our way, smiling indulgently at the enthusiastic little girl in the brightly striped hair scarf who was tugging her apologetic mother to the head of the queue to disembark. Lucy clattered down the noisy steel steps and virtually ran in to the airport lounge. A quick look around the busy terminal, her little head swivelling left to right, back to the left. Her search for her father was unsuccessful and disappointing.

'There's no one here for us, no one's waiting for me,' she whispered through quivering lips, her eyes full of hurt. I hid my own anger.

'Don't worry, Luce. Your dad will be finding a place to park. He must be here somewhere.'

I was furious and just about to call Yorgos when the twins bounded in to the Arrivals hall. Tony and Sam helped their father with our bags and we were bundled in to our old Volkswagen combi van, which months before I had noticed rusting beside Yorgos' workshop.

I didn't have a lot to say to Yorgos during the 20-minute drive to the Old Town, but suddenly thought of the boxes I had sent by ferryboat two days previously. I turned to look over my shoulder into the back of the van. There were no boxes.

'Did you manage to pick up all the things from the ferryboat this morning?' I asked.

Yorgos ran his hand through his hair, lips pursed together in a twisting motion. 'Oh God. The boat. I forgot all about that.'

That spelt the end of any attempt at conversation. I tried to focus my thoughts on the hotels and holidaymakers that seemed a bright contrast to the more mundane surroundings of our temporary Athens home.

My spirits were sinking fast.

As Yorgos pulled up outside the house I knew I really didn't want to go inside. The garden was a mess; my little home was in a similar state. I dumped the bags at the door and went straight to my neighbour's for a coffee. Lucy ran in to greet her godmother but didn't sit.

'Dad's taking me straight to Yiayia. Bye!' She was already pulling on Yorgos' arm, tugging him towards the door.

———

I finished my coffee and returned to my house. For a moment I was alone. I was tired, drained and on the verge of tears.

A knock on the door and Chris was at the window.

'Gidday there.' She was laughing as she and her friends moved into the sitting room. Through hugs I started to apologise for the state of the house.

'What the hell? Who cares about that? Come on Coll, relax! You're home, no more hospitals for a while. We've just seen Lucy with her dad and she looks great, so cheer up. Come on, we're taking you out. We've already ordered drinks next door, so let's go.'

So we did. We went to the restaurant next door, where we sat for hours enjoying local wine and the good home cooking of the Langanis family.

———

During the first few days back on Rhodes I tried to do everything; arrange to have a friend give Lucy her injection, ensure her Hickman was clean and okay and that she was eating properly at her grandmother's, clean and get the house in order, desperately try to catch up on everything with the boys, sort my things out, do all the national insurance paperwork, see everyone from work … In reality I achieved very little. The house remained a mess and the boys were wild, not used to having their freedom curbed by what they considered a nagging mother.

At the national insurance office I faced another barrier. Most of the paperwork from the hospitals in Athens was in order but the system refused to pay the large radiotherapy bill without another document from Saint Savas.

Lucy remained at her grandmother's apartment and I visited every day to check and change her Hickman. She always made it clear that she was glad to see the back of me. My friend Despina, a nurse who had grown up in Australia, had settled in to a routine with Lucy's injection on alternate days during the week and I was considering returning to work. Chris persuaded me to delay that by one day and I joined her and the girls on a trip to Lindos.

On the beach I spoke with John, who quickly talked me into skiing. The raft was busy with young holidaymakers, many of whom looked surprised when John's assistant unzipped the cover of his new monoski.

He handed me the ski, quickly squirting a drop of dishwashing liquid into the tight boot binding before I pulled it on and dropped off the side of the skiing platform. I'd almost forgotten the feeling moments before skiing and then on the water. Holding the right position as John turned the boat, waiting for the ski rope to tighten, there was that twinge of excitement/dread that hit my stomach; a fleeting thought of possible failure as I nodded to John. His powerful MasterCraft sped off towards the middle of Lindos Bay. Then that marvelous feeling of coming up out of the water, leaning back on the ski to give a powerful spray, the knowledge that yes, I was up and away.

Minutes later, I returned to the raft, embarrassed by the applauding spectators. John just smirked and told his next customer that I had taught him what he knew many years ago, adding with a smile and raised eyebrows that I still owed him a bottle of champagne for his first successful attempt to monoski.

I joined John in the ski boat for a couple of rounds. He asked about Lucy, and wanted all the details about how she was. I assured him she was looking much better than when he had seen her in Athens.

He said, 'By the way, have you checked your bank account lately?'

I was taken aback for a moment. 'No, not for a while. Why?'

'Oh, no reason really, I just wondered.' He kissed me on the cheek, waved to the girls and returned to his ski boat, quickly roaring off to tow three kids on inflatable ringos out of the bay.

Leaving the small beach, we trudged up the hill to the town to find other friends from England, Natalie and her parents, Rena and Cliff. The family had moved to Lindos in the mid-1980s to establish a restaurant and bar on the small beach. They'd recently relocated their Sunburnt Arms to the village centre, and we enjoyed a long cold spritzer in the cozy little pub.

Cliff, an ex-professional footballer, was his usual affable self. 'Hello, my dear. How's that little girl of ours? I hope she is doing better now than when John saw her. Heavens, we started worrying all over again then.'

'She's looking good,' I assured him, adding that I had left her in Rhodes knowing that she would want to get into the water in Lindos. 'It's difficult, Cliff. It's so hot and with the Hickman she knows she can't go anywhere near the water. It would have been like a torture, a punishment bringing her here.'

'Shame, John would have loved seeing her looking better. Amazing what he did for you guys, eh, Coll?'

'What did he do?' I asked.

'Oh, Gawd, typical of me to put my foot in it!' Cliff looked across the bar for support from his wife and daughter, who both lifted their eyebrows. They were saying nothing, so Cliff continued.

'Well, I may as well tell you 'cause you'll hear it from someone else anyway. After seeing you and Lucy in the hostel, John arrived in Lindos to start skiing again. He told us how poorly Lucy had looked, described her burnt little face, how tiny she was, how thin and tired you were. He talked about Athens all the time and kept asking what he could do to help. Well, in the end he came up with the idea to have a Lucy Day on the raft. He arranged for a champion skier he knows to "perform". John charged people to go on the raft and whatever money he made that day he put into your bank account.'

What? I was gob smacked, even more so when Natalie added, 'And I know how much he banked because he gave the 2,000 Euros to me to put in the account.'

Shocked, I started to cry, unable to curb the tears as I realised, yet again, what wonderful supportive friends I have.

Monday 24 June

Monday morning, the start of a new week and I feel I am finally getting myself and Lucy sorted out. Despina was here before 10am to give Lucy her injection. I changed the Hickman, gave her the usual 'stay out of the sun' warning and headed to the shop. I felt out of synch because it wasn't busy and I wasn't needed. My thoughts weren't on jewellery and making a sale. I was wondering what Lucy would be doing and if she was okay.

I talked with Michalis and, to the benefit of both I believe, we agreed that I should work three days a week (the busy ones when there are more than four cruise ships in the harbour) until Lucy and I return from her Athens check-up.

With Elena's 40-day memorial service just days away, I decided to visit Artemis and Tula. My decision to tell Lucy about her little friend's death a few days after she had passed away had, for some reason, amazed most of my friends in Elpida. They did not want their children to know that one of their friends had died and had warned me to be careful not to mention Elena's death near their children. Some were downright angry with me for telling Lucy, but I believed the children knew more than they let on and it was their right to know what was happening to their friends.

Artemis called and we decided to meet. Lucy was not going to be left at home so we headed off together to find Artemis and Tula in their spacious home in Coskinou village, just minutes from Rhodes town. They met us at the front door, the pretty mother and aunt now in black mourning clothes. The girls were full of smiles, fussing over Lucy, talking about her clothes, her slowly growing hair.

'Wow, your hair is amazing Lucy, it's growing back really well,' Tula said.

'I had a good hairdresser in TAO.' Lucy's quick reply had the girls laughing. The questions and answers continued non-stop. This wasn't the Lucy that most of her friends in Rhodes had seen so far. She wasn't reserved; there were no fleeting images of a little girl out of her depth. She didn't have to explain anything to Artemis and Tula, she knew that they knew and that was it. Lucy was totally at home in their company and didn't miss a beat when Artemis' polite, shy teenage son joined us in the kitchen.

'Lucy, this is Elena's big brother, Thodoris. Thodoris, this is the Loukia Lucy we've told you about. She had a very special friendship with your sister. She's one very special little girl.'

Thodoris smiled at Lucy, looking at her with sad, troubled eyes that wordlessly described his pain at meeting a young girl when he had just lost his sister to cancer. He was about to sit down when a man's voice called from elsewhere in the house.

'That's Dad,' he said, 'he'll want to meet you as well Lucy.' He strode off and returned seconds later with Artemis' husband on his arm.

Artemis had told me that her husband suffered from multiple sclerosis, a chronic disease that attacks the central nervous system. I had assumed he was mobile and was shocked to realise he was suffering so badly with the disease. Stavros was helped into a seat near the kitchen door and quickly focused on Lucy.

'So this is the Loukia I have heard so much about,' he said with difficulty. 'Well, welcome to our home Loukia. It is my pleasure to meet you and your mother.' He had a warm smile and was apologetic for his disability. Lucy was all smiles and immediately won yet another male fan.

We were treated to drinks, cakes and chocolates and, while Lucy chatted, I took in the surroundings, wondering if my daughter had noticed the kitchen. Little Elena was everywhere: photos with her mother, at the seaside, with other children at a playground, one startling image of Elena in a beautiful deep blue dress. She was a happy smiling little girl – an angel only lent.

It was unbearably sad, heart wrenching. Eyes smarting with tears, I blinked myself back to the conversation before the girls could read my thoughts. Vowing to be a frequent visitor to this sad home, I told Lucy it was time for us to go. Tula was the first to move, going into the lounge to return with a large, pink carton in her arms.

'This is for you Lucy. I know how much you like Barbie and I heard you talking about a Barbie house in TAO. Well, this is a special one because it's a radio as well.'

Lucy was gracious, hugging Artemis and Tula, turning back to kiss Stavros on the cheek.

'Wow, this can be from Elena,' she said, struggling to hold the oversized package. Her comment ended the bright chatter and crumbled the façade of happy smiles we had built over the hour of conversation in the kitchen.

In a farewell hug with Artemis I totally lost it. All the bottled up feelings suddenly surfaced as we clung to one another. I can't imagine Artemis' pain, her loss. She is incredibly brave, but I wonder what lies behind that wonderful smile she puts on for Lucy.

Sunday 30 June

Elpida has lost another child. Gone is little Eleni, who had been battling against all odds in intensive care. I want to call her parents but I can't, I'm a coward.

Since our return to Rhodes, keeping Lucy happy and occupied has been a struggle. Her friends visit her if she is in the Old Town with her grandmother during the day, but when they inevitably head off to the beach Lucy, who can't stay out in the hot mid-summer sun for long and can't go swimming, is left unhappy and disgruntled. She is fed up with television and, because alternatives were few, I bought her a Playstation. I hate it but at least it puts a smile on her face and keeps her indoors, away from the sun.

In the evenings we go to Calithea, a beautiful area on the east coast of Rhodes. Once a health spa, its waters attracted the Mediterranean's wealthiest travellers, but now it has fallen into neglect, only a shadow of its former glory remaining. As a swimming area, however, its cool, clear waters are unmatched and in the evenings it is quieter than many other areas on the island. Lucy paddles in the shallow waters but even then I'm afraid of her splashing or tripping over and soaking the Hickman.

I watch Lucy watching other children jumping, diving and swimming, her face often sad and lonely. I understand her anger and her sadness. There is no way out, she knows why she had the Hickman and she knows she can't swim. End of story.

The Playstation is a temporary solution to the problem.

I decided not to show Lucy the notice for Elena's memorial service and that I would go without reminding her. However, Lucy was too quick for me. I was on the telephone when she saw the small black and white photograph of her little friend. She went straight to my sewing box, grabbed the scissors, cut the piece out of the newspaper and very quickly added it to a wooden frame on her desk.

'When is Elena's service, Mum?'

'It's early tomorrow morning.' I winced, trying to find a quick reason why Lucy should not accompany me to the service.

'Luce, I know you know about Elena's death, but you know what so many of the Greek people are like, they don't expect to see children at funerals and well, it could be difficult if ...'

Lucy cut me short, I didn't need to finish. 'I don't want to go tomorrow, Mum. There'll be too many people there and I don't want them all looking at me. Can we go tonight? I want to see where Elena is. We can get her some flowers, eh Mum?'

'Good idea.'

I called Artemis and arranged to go to Coskinou later in the evening. As we reached the car, Lucy said, 'Wait a minute, Mum. I want to take something else to Elena.' She ran back to the house and returned with one of her favourite cartoon characters, a pink and white Minnie Mouse. It was a small plastic figurine, nothing special, but one of her treasures nevertheless.

The cemetery, just a quick drive away from Artemis' home, was in typical Greek Orthodox style. There were rows of large, marble tombs, headed with crosses and decorated with fresh and plastic flowers. More accustomed to flat memorial plaques set in lawns, I have always found these cemeteries overwhelming.

Elena's grave was probably one of the cemetery's largest. It was a canopied pink marble bed and dressing table, with masses of pink and white rosebuds, plants, butterflies and a beautiful porcelain doll, basically anything to make Elena's resting place pretty and childlike. I was taken aback by it. Lucy was fine, helping Artemis carefully to place the large white daisies for the following morning's service and giving her lost friend the little cartoon character.

Only then was Lucy quiet. Only then were we all reminded of her link with Elena.

Artemis touched my arm. 'Lucy will never forget my little girl, you know.'

I couldn't speak.

'Thanks for coming tonight, Lucy,' Artemis said as we walked back to my car. 'You will always be someone very special in this family, you know that, don't you?'

Leaning on the window and looking across the car's front she smiled, mouthing, 'Thank you so much.'

'You will come in the morning, won't you?' she said to me as we pulled away. 'Of course,' I promised.

The drive home was difficult.

'Mum, will Elena come back to Earth?' 'No,' I said, 'she's an angel now, a very special little angel.'

'Why did she have to die?' 'I don't know.'

'Do you remember Elena telling her mum to shut up? Mum, do you remember? We all laughed. Wouldn't it be nice if she could do that now? Do you think she's in Paradise, Mum?' 'Probably.'

'If I pray hard enough maybe she'll come back.' 'No, I don't think so Lucy.'

A long pause. 'Okay then, she's going to be my angel,' Lucy said, turning to gaze out the window, lost in thoughts that I didn't dare interrupt.

Lucy's moods seesawed, easygoing, chirpy and bright one minute and totally the opposite the next. There was no in-between. I put it down to a combination of the Rebif injections, the heat and Lucy's inability to relax, play or swim normally.

Every day I tried to sneak off for a swim, a quick dip to cool down. How did Lucy cool down and relax?

Many times she was miserable and cried.

'I hate it. I hate those injections; I hate this Hickman, I hate the heat and not being able to swim. I hate it all!'

She even said she wished she could die.

'Why can't I just die, Mum? That would be a lot easier. Why do I have to go through all of this?'

If I tried to hug and comfort her she pulled away, angry and dejected.

I had no answers for her. What could I say other than to remind her of what her specialists had said? How should I tell an eight year-old to be patient, to understand that she was one of the lucky children? She was still alive.

After all those months, I realised I had no real answers.

Wednesday 10 July

Lucy and I returned to Athens last night. After an easy flight and transfer we were back to a quiet Elpida in a room on the third floor. Smaro was quick to find us; we chatted and then went to KETH to see Effy and Yorgos. He hasn't been at all well, with nosebleeds and sickness after his chemotherapy coupled with a bad reaction to a blood platelet transfusion.

Yorgos was thin, wide-eyed and pale. Effy wasn't much better. Both looked shattered and I wondered how they would cope with any further therapies. Back at Elpida Lucy and I slept well. It was strange to be back. Even though the room was sterile and soulless without personal touches, it was almost like being home again. I felt safe there, quite the opposite of my feeling in Rhodes.

This morning we were into TAO at 8.30am courtesy of the minibus. We were its only passengers so I thought the clinic would be quiet. Far from it. The waiting room was already busy and the clinic was packed with new children. It was depressing.

We've been away from TAO for one month. When we left it seemed the clinic was emptying and somehow I believed it would stay that way. I was wrong. Cancer doesn't stop. It takes a breather now and again, and then it's off again to find more victims.

Lucy was called for a blood test and led away by a bubbly microbiologist named Effy.

'Mum can stay here, eh Lucy? We girls have a lot of catching up to do. Now, tell me, what's happening on Rhodes? What about that friend of your brothers you were telling me about last month ...'

———

I was delighted to see that Papadakis was in the outpatients' office that morning. He assured us that Lucy's results were good.

'And you're looking good – must be that great climate on Rhodes, Lucy. I was there a couple of years ago with Artemis and little Elena. Great place, fantastic beaches, the seawater is unmatched. You agree Lucy?'

When he mentioned the sea, Lucy's pert, happy face altered. Her specialist noticed it straight away.

'What's wrong? What did I say?' Lucy just looked at him.

'Go on, tell me. You were as bright as a button a few seconds ago and now you're ready to cry. Are you in pain?'

'No.' Lucy lowered her head.

Her specialist glanced at me enquiringly, and then back at Lucy.

'What's wrong then, Lucy? How can I help you if I don't know what's troubling you?'

Lucy lifted her head, met his eyes and held them. 'I can't go for a swim, that's what's wrong!'

Her outburst was unexpected and it left her doctor a picture of surprise and bemusement.

'Oh ... well now I know where the problem lies, let's see if we can fix it. Any problems with your Hickman, Lucy?'

'No, the stupid pipe is fine. That's the reason I can't swim. Because Mum is always so worried about getting it wet. She takes me to the beach in the evening and let's me paddle like a little child. I know it's not her fault but I hate the Hickman. I hate being like this. You sent us back to Rhodes but I would be better off here. At least in Athens I don't want to go swimming.'

Papadakis smiled kindly. 'Now I know what you're feeling Lucy. You're back on Rhodes so close to that wonderful tantalising water and you can't go in. Like we're punishing you after all you've been through.'

Her specialist stopped, ran his right hand across his chin in a pensive movement and looked at us. He was up in a flash, out from behind his desk and through the door. He returned quickly, his white coat swinging. Holding the door open, he held his hand out for Lucy. 'Dr Haidas wants to see you.'

Lucy rather reluctantly took his hand and I followed them into the director's office, where he quickly checked her neck and her hands.

'You're right,' he said looking at the younger doctor. 'It's a sin, a shame to torture her.' Bending down to look Lucy in the eye he added, 'Is that how you feel Lucy, when you can't join your friends swimming?'

She nodded, said nothing.

Haidas looked at her again then turned towards her specialist. 'You're right. The Hickman can go.'

Lucy looked at me. I looked at her. We were both wondering if we had heard correctly.

'It will mean staying on in Athens for a few days. Lucy could come back in tomorrow and I'll check for surgery time for Friday or Monday. Can you stay in Athens that long?'

I didn't have to consider the answer.

'Of course, another few days won't make any difference,' I assured him.

Lucy looked a different girl. With a dazzling smile, she seemed to float out of the office and into the waiting room. News always travelled fast on TAO so within seconds everyone was smiling. The clinic invariably needed and always appreciated good news.

Lucy bounded out of the hospital and skipped along the street to Elpida, in a hurry to share her news with her friends. I left her with Maria, another child who had been battling illness for a long time, and ran to Saint Savas to change the papers relating to Lucy's radiation treatment.

That, as usual, was a performance. Once again I was struck by how difficult and complicated the paper trail was. I was sure it could be streamlined. Zampaties was not available but fortunately I found his smiling secretary, who could not have been more helpful. I noted quickly that the new paper revealed that Lucy had undergone more than 70 radiation sessions; a mind-boggling total for an eight year-old.

From that hospital I ran off to the IKA hospital to arrange Lucy's

Rebif prescription and, typically, straight in to another struggle with a snooty doctor who complained about my not having an appointment. I pointed out it wasn't easy to make an appointment when you didn't know from one day to the next what was going to happen to your child.

She just looked at me. I changed tactic.

'Look, I know you're extremely busy. I've noticed that the chairs in that waiting room outside never seem to empty. And I realise I don't have an appointment but I didn't know I had to arrange that before leaving Rhodes. No one took the time to explain this system to me. It's crazy that I have to run from one hospital to the other, knowing that I will now have to go to an IKA office to have your prescription authorised and then go to the IKA pharmacy.

'Normally I would only be here for a day and that would be even worse for me timewise. But today my daughter was surprised with good news. She's probably having surgery to take out her Hickman the day after tomorrow, so if this really is such a problem I will go to the office and try to make an appointment for Friday and then hope like hell I will be able to get everything done before we return to Rhodes to the rest of my family.'

I took a breath, realising I had rattled that off pretty rapidly. I was angry, frustrated and fed up. I stood up to leave the office and the well-coiffed brunette with piercing blue eyes relented. 'Okay, I didn't realise you were from Rhodes,' she said apologetically, handing over a quickly scribbled prescription.

'Thanks, much appreciated,' I told her as I moved towards the door.

'I wish your daughter a full recovery.' A long sigh before she added, 'And please call in the next patient on your way out.'

Lucy had found company at Elpida. She was entertaining a quiet and withdrawn Dimitri, who I believed was smiling behind the green surgery mask that covered so much of his wonderful little face. I talked with Smaro – ah, what a great lady, another special friend – and we both heard that Antony and his parents were expected back at the hostel in the morning. Lucy and Dimitri were delighted but Smaro and I knew that his unplanned visit was in no way good news.

Friday 12 July

Yesterday I left Lucy snoozing at the hostel (Smaro said she would check on her) and hurried in to Syntagma early to run some chores for Michalis for the shop. I then wandered to IKA's central pharmacy to get Lucy's Rebif prescription. It was so much easier than the first time. I knew exactly where to go (stairs, long corridors), what to have with me (the necessary ice packs and an insulated bag to ensure the medication remained refrigerated) and what to expect (it amazed and worried me that the queue at that pharmacy for restricted medication was long and constant). I wanted to cry.

The afternoon and evening were spent with friends at Elpida. Lucy was with Dimitri when Antony joined them in the dining room. He made such a fuss of Lucy, who glowed under the 17 year-old's flirtatious gaze. 'I think I've found my wife to be,' he said. 'What do you think Lucy? I reckon we'd make a good pair. You'll just have to promise me you won't look at any of those good-looking boys on Rhodes and I'll wait for you to grow up a bit. We'll have a big island wedding. It will be like a TAO reunion and you and all our friends will be well again. You'll be the most beautiful bride in the world and Dimitri can be our best man. What do you think Dimitri?'

The younger boy had fallen silent. 'We'll see who Luce chooses when the time comes. Then we'll see who will be the groom and who will be the best man!' he said.

'Ah, I have a challenge here,' Antony laughed. He reached across and hugged both Lucy and Dimitri in a way that had us all fighting to hold back tears. Antony was grinning, at Lucy, at me and at his mother who returned his smile, but turned quickly to wipe away telltale tears before they spilled down her cheeks.

'What's wrong?' I asked, noting Smaro's happy face was also marked by concern.

'Nothing so far, but the doctors are worried that Antony's temperature is never normal. There's always something showing in his blood tests. I know it's wrong, but whenever he talks of the future I just lose it. I wonder if he has a future; I wonder how much longer he will have to live under the threat of this bloody illness. I wonder …'

Pagona turned away, leaving us struggling for words.

Lucy lost her Hickman today, after a long wait at the clinic. We'd gone to TAO early for her injection and her specialist suggested that the line could be removed using local anesthetic, but Lucy was not having it. She was adamant, so we had to wait until late afternoon when Papadakis could find time in the obviously busy schedule in the operating theatre.

Lucy was a hungry and impatient outpatient as she eyed and described everything she could not eat until the quick surgery was performed.

Afterwards there were no moans, even her hunger was forgotten, as we waited for any side effects of the anesthetic to wear off, and then headed back to the hostel.

It was quiet and there was no sign of Dimitri and Antony, who we heard later were both having tests at the bone marrow outpatients clinic. I called the boys' mothers and spoke to Effy, who assured me that Yorgos was much stronger and brighter.

Lucy still found company at the hostel, something that a late finishing 'big' Dimitri remarked on. 'That's the Lucy we all miss. She has the ability to brighten everyone's day. Look at her, that little girl rarely speaks to anyone and Lucy already has her playing. Amazing. We could do with her here more often, but of course that's something I would never wish on her. The less we see of her, the better for Lucy,' he added with a smile, kissing Lucy on the top of her head. 'See you for her next tests?'

'Yes, we'll be back in a month for a scan,' I told him as my mobile buzzed.

It was Pam, one of the founding members of the Make A Wish foundation in Greece.

'Hello Colleen. I've got good news. We've got the go-ahead for Lucy's wish. Her doctors think she can make the trip as long as you can guarantee that she will take her medication. All we have to think about now is arranging everything. I need you to get the passports ready and anything you pay for just let me know. You won't have to pay anything.'

I was taken aback and wanted to ask questions but Pam said she was busy. 'Don't worry. I'll be in touch. Bye for now and love to Lucy.'

With that the line went dead. I was left standing in the Elpida playroom, staring at my mobile.

'Mum, what's wrong?'

'Nothing, nothing at all. Just a wish about to come true ...' Lucy looked at me as if I was talking gibberish.

'That was Make A Wish. You're going to see Nana and you're taking your brothers with you.'

What a shame I didn't have a camera ready to capture the look on Lucy's face! Delight, wonder, bliss. All rolled into one, huge smile.

Lucy is asleep now, tucked into my side. She still looks happy.

God how I wish she always looked like this.

Saturday 13 July

We flew back to Rhodes early this morning and Lucy woke her brothers. She bounded into their bedroom, literally bouncing on to their beds.

'Yanni, wake up!'

Yanni sat up in a fright, looking at his sister, shaking his head as if to leave whatever dream she had interrupted behind him. 'Hey Lucy, how did it go in Athens? Your tests okay?'

'Oh, they were fine. Look,' she said, pulling up her t-shirt, 'my Hickman has gone. I don't have that stupid plug anymore. And guess what?'

Yanni was just about making sense of his sister's quick words, which had also woken the twins.

'We're going to see Nana. My wish is going to come true. We're all going to Nana.'

Lucy climbed into bed with Yanni and the four talked and laughed about the prospect of going to New Zealand.

'Oh, we'll have to speak English. New Zealandish,' Sam quipped, 'like Mum does when she's on the phone with Nana.'

I didn't want to break the spell so I moved into the living room to call Pat and moments later my mother. 'Mum, we're coming home with Make A Wish.'

'That will be nice dear! What day will you be here? You know I have bowls on Thursday and get my hair done on Friday – you'd better make it early in the week.'

'Mum, we'll be there for nearly two weeks.'

Silence at the other end of the phone.

'Oh dear, what will I do then? You can't stay here. Heavens where will you all stay?'

I laughed and assured my mother that something would be arranged. She was right though – four children and a mother would be a bit of a handful for the trip organisers.

Strangely enough, Pat came up with the solution a day later. She'd been talking with her neighbour, excited at the prospect of the trip, although a little daunted by the possibility of having us all in a caravan in her backyard.

'I'd hardly finished speaking and Doug said, "Hang on a sec, Pat. Let me just have a word with Barbara." He rushed across our shared driveway into his house, and was back outside within seconds. He was beaming. "Knew it. Barbara's agreed. Coll and her family can have our granny house for as long as they are in Christchurch. What do you think of that? Just the thing I'd say! Might need a bit of a cleanup 'cause no one has lived in there since my mother passed away. Of course the kids don't need to know that do they? We'll have it as right as rain by the time Coll gets here! Just put the idea to Coll and see how she feels." What do you think? I know you've only seen photos of our house, but this little granny house is right next door. It could be perfect, it would be like staying with Trish and me but you and the kids will have your privacy as well.'

I was flabbergasted at Doug's generosity, assured my sister that her neighbour was a godsend and phoned Pam at Make A Wish. I explained Pat's neighbour's offer and Pam was delighted.

Another step on our way to Lucy's wish.

21

Thursday 15 August

Ridiculous – a month has passed and I haven't put pen to paper. Good or bad thing, I don't know. I guess I don't feel the burning need to express my feelings as I did during the months in Athens when this notebook was my sounding board. My friends are never far away so I talk to them and find most of my worries and fears are not so daunting once I have talked them over.

I am like Lucy, good some days and 'off' others. We've had a month without the Hickman, a month of high points, laughter, celebrations, and a return to something closer to our normal life, with a return to working full-time. And of course there have been some low spots.

I wonder if our lives will ever be the same.

Life with Lucy without the Hickman was a lot easier. On our return to Rhodes I had to change the dressing following her surgery. As always, Lucy was pretty awful the first time I touched the dressing but we got over that and just counted the days until the small wound had closed properly and she could swim again.

I had continued our almost daily trips to Calithea and other nearby beaches, letting Lucy paddle, still careful not to wet the dressing. It was like a ten-day countdown to the evening when we went to the main beach in Rhodes town. I had finished work at 6pm and found Lucy, already wearing her bikini, waiting for me in the garden, a small bag by her side, with a new Barbie towel. She was happy and excited, talking non-stop as we drove through the busy early evening traffic to park near the casino on Elli Beach.

I locked my car, took Lucy's hand and we walked down a few steps on to the beach. Suddenly Lucy stopped, pulling on my hand desperately. I turned to face her, thinking that she had left something in the car. She was holding her beach bag in front of her, her head down, chin almost on her chest.

'What's wrong? Have we forgotten something?' She shook her head, pulling at the small pink scarf she has tied over her short hair.

'Come on then. Let's swiiiiim!' Her head went down even further, so I bent down to see what was wrong. Lucy was sobbing, silently.

'What's up?' She continued to stare down at the beach bag she clutched with both hands.

'I'm not going in. Everyone will stare at me. They'll see the scars from the Hickman and on my neck. They'll see my horrible hair. I'm not swimming.'

I touched her arm, thinking I could help her, thinking I could change her mind. I was wrong. Lucy was suddenly vicious.

'Get away from me!' she hissed. 'Take me home. I don't want to swim. I can't go in the water. I don't want to be anywhere near you. Take me home,' she demanded.

We returned to the car. Lucy had stopped crying but remained angry and aggressive. I was close to tears, not knowing what to do.

'Come on, Luce, it can't be that bad. Let's go somewhere else. I know you want to swim, you've been waiting for this for so long.'

'Don't talk to me. Take me home! Now!'

I drove back along the busy Mandrake Parade, past the moored pleasure and day-trip boats, in and out of the Old Town to the colourful fishing boat marina, and on towards the main commercial harbor near our entrance, into what was once the Jewish area of the Old Town. The closer we got to the house the more aggressive Lucy became. She was beside herself, screaming.

'I don't want to go anywhere! I don't ever want to go to the beach again!'

I didn't know what to do and had no idea how to handle the situation.

I was lost. What should have been one of the happiest moments of the summer had turned into a disaster. My mobile buzzed; it was Sharon.

'I'm going for a swim,' she said. 'Wanna join me?'

'You're a godsend. Yes, I do want to swim but I need to talk to you. Let me take Lucy home first. Where shall I meet you?' Sharon suggested Zefiros, the east coast beach that was popular with locals.

'Okay, I'll be there in five minutes,' I told her and signalled to turn into the Old Town.

'Don't you dare!' Lucy cried. 'You're not taking me home. You're not going anywhere without me!'

So I continued towards Zefiros on the other side of town, pulling up behind Sharon's car on the road between the beach and Rhodes' main cemetery. Sharon was surprised to see Lucy but, reading my face, said nothing. 'Hello Lucy. I didn't know you were coming as well.'

'I'm not. I'll sit in the car until Mum finishes.'

'Oh, it's too hot for that. At least come on down and wait on the sand. Come on Lucy.' Lucy accepted Sharon's extended hand and they walked together on to the sandy beach.

'You know what you're missing, Lucy. You know you want to feel that water around you again. Come on, let's just run in. Quick, throw your bag down here with mine; Mum too. Let's drop everything here. Take a breath and here we go! Run in and don't stop!'

And we did just that. Suddenly we were in the water, splashing, laughing, all that anger, frustration and anguish gone from Lucy's little face. She laughed, diving and swimming under the water. When she finally collapsed on the sand she was glowing.

Thanks Sharon for being there then, for calling at the right time. Now Lucy and I swim every evening and it's wonderful.

We had an end-of-Hickman party in our garden in the Old Town. Lucy invited her school friends and they feasted on pizza, pies and cakes. They played musical chairs, statues, and pin-the-tail-on-the-elephant (thanks Sam, for the great drawing). Very few knew what we were celebrating but that didn't matter; what did matter was Lucy's happy, carefree smile. It was as if the months and Athens and those vicious treatments had never touched her.

The Make A Wish trip was never far from my mind. Pam called me many times; firstly to ensure that I had started to get the passports sorted and secondly to arrange flights. The paperwork was time-consuming, especially as I had returned to work daily at the shop. Documents had to be completed early in the morning, or through the travel agency I used to finalise the passports once I had permission from Yorgos to take the children (all minors) out of Greece. Yanni already had a passport, obtained when he had visited Hungary to represent Greece in kayaking championships a couple of years previously.

Actually, he'd been a bit of a worry since receiving his national exam results. He was withdrawn and moody until an English friend (another Chris) invited him to go the England for a holiday. Chris had seen the change in Yanni, who was always bright and comfortable in her company. He had become quiet and introverted.

Yanni didn't say no to Chris' offer, although he was a bit reluctant when she was unable to get him on her flight back to the UK. She found a cheap alternative that would arrive at Gatwick around the same time as her flight. A few days later I was helping him check in at Rhodes Airport. Yanni was looking good in a new white shirt and trendy jeans. He was a picture of confidence and he had a big smile for the pretty little blonde behind the check-in desk.

Monday 19 August

It's Monday evening and I am alone in a quiet house, alone with my thoughts, which are anything but positive.

Little Dimitri is back in the clinic. I've known for several days now and still can't believe it.

I called Smaro a couple of days ago. She told me that Dimitri was fine, although he had a temperature, adding that it was probably something to do with his Hickman as it was red and sore looking. That apart, she said, he was eating more and seemed to be getting stronger.

The next day Antony's mum's name came up on my mobile phone

caller-ID. I was at the shop and moved out on to the side of the store to talk. It was Antony on the phone.

'Hi Mum,' he said with a chuckle. 'How's my wife to be?' I assured him that his young admirer was fine and I scoffed at his comment that he would lose his little lady to a local lad. 'Not likely!'

'Whew, I can relax again then! Take care Colleen, here's Mum.' I knew straight away that something was wrong.

'What is it? What's wrong with Tony?'

'It's not Tony,' she said. 'It's Dimitri. He and Smaro are back in the clinic. Ah, that's what I have heard and I can't bring myself to call her. I can't find the strength. Dimitri had a temperature and I'm dying with worry as Antony always has a slight temperature.'

'Put the phone down,' I told her. 'I'll call Smaro and see what's happening.'

I clicked off and walked back in to the shop. Numb, hardly thinking, I was seeing only Dimitri's face, lit up with his wide smile, his little eyes sparkling. No, the disease couldn't have returned, I told myself. It couldn't possibly do that again. I called Smaro's number and said, 'Hi, where are you guys?'

A sigh.

'Ah, my lovely friend, we are back in the clinic. It's back. The temperature wasn't from the Hickman. It's back, it's back.'

I didn't know what to say. What could I say? We'd been through so much together. You can't touch someone through a telephone but I closed my eyes and hugged Smaro. I couldn't speak, I couldn't tell her what I was trying to do but I knew she felt it.

It was all I could do.

Today Lucy and I notched up another milestone. Despina, who had been giving Lucy her injections, left on holiday and I had to take over. I tossed and turned all night. What little sleep I did have was broken by a recurring dream of holding Lucy's arm, jabbing the needle in, her screams.

I was up early, before she could see me practising as the TAO nurses had shown me, injecting an orange. I must have run to the toilet four or five times before it was time for Lucy to surface.

It was like the first Hickman change only worse. I was scared of hurting her and dreaded her moans and screams. Lucy was reluctant to sit down but did, on a small stool near the kitchen door.

I took the injection from its protective casing, carefully syringed the oily medication from the tiny phial, removed the needle and tapped the syringe to dislodge any air bubbles. Trying to control my shaking hand, I slowly pressed the plunger to expel any air bubbles through the needle until I saw a drop of medicine on the tip. Holding the injection in my right hand, I wiped the outside of the top of Lucy's right arm with an alcohol swab, squeezed the skin slightly and inserted the needle.

Lucy didn't move; she didn't squeal and she didn't cringe. I depressed the plunger and slowly emptied the barrel then removed the needle.

It was that easy. All over in a matter of seconds. And, guess what? Lucy said she didn't feel anything. I went off to work a different person, light headed and elated, realising that concern and stress over arranging Lucy's injections at the hospital during our stay in Christchurch had been premature. I was minus one worry.

Friday 23 August

Lucy and I are back on Rhodes after two nights in Athens for a scheduled scan and blood tests. It's hard to describe my feelings, which range from unbound happiness and hope to a sadness that is so raw it is almost beyond words.

Flying to Athens and moving yet again back into Elpida was an effortless routine. I was happy that Lucy took everything in her stride; she was confident travelling and even more self-assured in her conversations with the hostel staff and her doctors.

Elpida was busy and Dimitri apologised for putting us in a small room with a single bed. That didn't matter; we've had many months of sharing a single bed. Lucy's only friend there was Maria, whose petite mother Yorgia welcomed us with endless cups of coffee and tales of all our friends. Effy and Yorgos had left for a break on Rhodes; Magda was in the surgical ward recovering from surgery; and both Dimitri and Antony were in TAO. It was a sobering start to our stay in Athens.

Lucy was scheduled for an early-morning scan and, for once, finished early. Walking up the flight of stairs from the x-ray and scan area we met Dr Papadakis. As usual he was in a hurry, but he spoke briefly to Lucy and told me to check with him just after midday for the results of the scan.

Lucy beamed. 'Great! That means I can catch up with all my friends in TAO!' Dr Papadakis ruffled the top of her head and touched me on the shoulder. 'That says it all, doesn't it? God, how these children feel for one another.'

He sighed and hurried off down the stairs leaving us to go and find Yorgia and Magda. Yorgia was sitting on an uncomfortable-looking chair at the side of the bed. She wasn't asleep but it was obvious that her thoughts were miles away. Magda was like a little crumpled puppet, her strings a mass of tubes connecting her not to chemo, but to other medication. She was asleep, a tiny broken bird on that big hospital bed. I bent to stop Lucy from approaching Yorgia but I wasn't quick enough; the flash of recognition and love on our friend's face was enough to tell me that we were meant to be there.

Hugs. Long hugs that expressed our feelings without any words. Little Magda stirred and woke with an angelic smile. 'Loukia! I knew you would come and see me.'

The little china doll came to life, her smile reaching into our hearts. I felt her joy at seeing her friend; the bond between Lucy and Magda was extraordinary. Lucy settled on the bed with Magda and Yorgia and I talked. Magda's specialists had decided on changes in her treatment; surgery was expected to quicken her recovery and their return to normal family life. I was thrilled but sensed a nagging doubt that Yorgia's eyes showed, but she did not express.

In TAO we found three of Lucy's favourite males: Alexandros, Antony and Dimitri.

Alexandros was in the waiting room with another young patient when Lucy walked into the clinic. He was chatting, talking quickly, and explaining something to the other boy who, unlike Alexandros, was not an outpatient. He was wired to medication hanging from the stand that the boisterous Alexandros seemed intent on tipping over, until a glare from a disapproving Eleni, the nurses' aide, stopped him in his tracks. It was then that he noticed Lucy.

'Luce!' Alexandros' face changed, his dazzling eyes matched only by his smile as he bounded across the waiting room to pull his friend into the ward. 'Let's go and find Antony. He'll be almost as pleased to see you as I am,' he said as the pair disappeared through the swinging doors. I expected to hear a shout from Eleni, but when I caught her eye she was shaking her head and smiling. So, she has a soft side after all, I thought.

I headed back out of the clinic to the steps and found Smaro, Pagona and Joanna deep in conversation over iced coffees. My three friends were starved of good news. Their children's futures remained threatened by dark clouds of doubt that only medicine and miracles could lift, yet all three women clung to threads of hope. We returned to TAO together, Smaro and Pagona to join their boys in the ward and Joanna to wrench Alexandros away from his friends.

'I'll be back in a few days!' Alexandros assured them, adding, 'And I'll see you when you get back from your grandmother. Don't forget Luce, we all want postcards!' As always, he seemed a boy much older than his eight years. Alexandros left us with his usual cheeky smile, and Lucy and I spent a few more minutes with Antony and Dimitri before heading to the waiting room to find Dr Papadakis.

<hr>

We pushed through the swing doors into the waiting room as he entered from the main entrance. He had the air of a man on a winning streak. Seeing us his face broke into a wide smile. In one movement he slammed Lucy's thick folder on the top of the reception desk and turned to meet my gaze.

'It's clear! Lucy's scan is clear!' The meticulous specialist was so happy he hugged us.

'What do you think of that then, Lucy? Looks like we've beaten him this time.'

It was a magical moment. Like a payment after all his (and everyone else's) hard work, all our worry and anguish, the clinic's knowledge and wisdom put to the test and … it all came off. Lucy's 50-50 odds were on the positive side. I returned to TAO later in the evening to talk again to her specialist. He was still ecstatic at the scan results, and spoke of the perfect timing of the Make A Wish trip that he had set in motion.

'It's perfect timing, like a celebration,' he said, handing me a handwritten statement detailing Lucy's cancer should I need it in New Zealand. We talked about carrying the Rebif injections throughout the journey.

'I've found a freezer bag that is just about the same size as the packet of injections. I'll just give them to the airline crew, as I always have to do flying back to Rhodes from here,' I said.

Papadakis was amused when I explained that the airlines, with stricter post-9/11 security, classed the injections as potentially dangerous weapons. 'Guard those injections with your life,' he said. 'I wish you and Lucy and your boys the trip of a lifetime, a trip to celebrate Lucy's life … and hey, don't forget to bring me back a New Zealand lamb!'

I left his office feeling light hearted and found Lucy deep in conversation with Antony, who was on medication again. He looked tired and sad, a shadow of the handsome young man who had entertained us so often at the hostel. Dimitri was asleep so Lucy kissed him gently on his forehead and we left the clinic to return to Elpida.

I didn't sleep well as I was struggling to come to terms with my feelings. On the one hand Lucy had managed to beat her cancer, beat it up; and on the other her precious friends were still fighting, boxers going the full distance knowing that all odds were against them.

When we arrived back on Rhodes, Effy was at the airport to pick us up. She and Yorgos were enjoying a few days at home, a much-needed break from the regimentation of the hostel and hospital visits, a breath of fresh air, family and old friends. Yorgos' doctor hadn't been keen on the trip considering his problems with nosebleeds and the need for immediate transfusions, and had made it clear that Effy would be held responsible if anything went wrong. Effy had called me just after Lucy's scan and said she would be at the airport. She was adamant, saying she had to talk to me.

We sped off towards Rhodes, Lucy and Yorgos chatting happily in the back of the car.

Effy started. She and her fragile little son had travelled from Athens to Rhodes by ship. Flying was out of the question as the cabin pressure could affect Yorgos and his nosebleeds, so Effy had booked a cabin on one of the large inter-island ferries. She was prepared for the boring 14-hour trip.

'Yorgos was fine when we left Athens. We ate in the ship's restaurant and went to bed rather early because I didn't want to keep Yorgos in the smoky public areas.

'Unusually we both drifted off to sleep quickly. Suddenly, Yorgos was shaking me awake. He was crying, pointing at the bed, which was covered in blood that was streaming from his nose. You know that's always my worst dread, the thing I fear the most whenever we are away from the hostel and the hospital,' she said, her eyes fixed on the road ahead, but her thoughts elsewhere.

'Yorgos was white, wide-eyed and panic stricken. I cursed myself for making the trip, knowing that something like this would happen. We were at sea, in the middle of who knows where, my son was losing blood, crying, shaking from fear and I didn't know what to do. I really didn't. I grabbed the bag I had with gauze pads and plugs, scrambling about to find anything to stop the blood.

'When I turned back towards Yorgos she was on the bed between us. Someone was there in the cabin with us.'

Effy stopped for a second, looked across at me, smiled, shrugged and continued.

'I gave Yorgos the pads and somehow there was this woman standing, hovering, I can't describe it really, between Yorgos and myself. She was dressed in black, all black like a shroud; I couldn't see her hands or feet. I just remember she had the most beautiful, serene face.

'Without moving her lips I heard her speak.

'"Don't worry Effy. Don't panic, my dear girl. Your child will be fine. I am here to look after you both. See, everything will be all right now."

'I can remember looking at the figure, blinking, thinking, this can't be happening, this can't be real. But she was there, I saw her, I heard her.' Effy took a deep breath and continued.

'I looked at Yorgos. He'd stopped crying. I moved slightly to pull the gauze away from his nose. The bleeding had stopped, his nose was clean; there was no sign of the bleeding, just a little dried blood on his nostrils.

'He was smiling and the woman had gone. "Yorgaki (little Yorgos) did you see her?" "See who Mum?"'

'It was weird. I remember an eerie calm, like everything was normal. And I wasn't scared, not at all. I didn't question anything. I just knew that she was there for us.

'Isn't that strange? It has to be the strangest thing I have ever experienced but, I promise you, it was real.'

Effy was driving fast – she always drives fast – while she was telling me her story.

'That's why I had to pick you up from the airport,' she said. 'I had to tell you, to see your face and your reaction.'

Had someone else told me the story I probably would have scoffed. I really wasn't into miracles lately, but this was Effy talking. Effy, my thin, trendy young friend. Effy, the straight talker. Fiery Effy, who was quick to anger but just as quick to forgive.

Effy didn't believe in tales and miracles either.

But this was her story and I believed her.

End of August

Lucy returned from Athens a different child, taking, it seems, everything in her stride. The injections are routine, although I still have to be patient and get her at the right moment. She's careful about staying in the sunshine and ventures out only in the late afternoon for swims with her friends. She looks confident again, more like my 'old' Lucy. Her hair is growing back and, although she still wears a hat or cap most of the time, she's not so conscious about it and quickly tells anyone who doesn't know any better that she was tired of long hair and had it all cut off!

I was making the last preparations for our trip. With passports, driver's licence and all our paperwork ready, Pam assured me that the travel arrangements were finalised. We would be flying with Singapore Airlines, with a day-long stopover in Singapore to break the long journey from Athens to Christchurch. All I needed to do was get my children and our clothes sorted out so everything would be ready for our early morning 2 September departure.

That was easier said than done. First move was to buy the set of luggage I'd always dreamed of, a set of bright red suitcases with a matching vanity (with a little mirror and pockets for the jars of make-up and creams that I very rarely use) that I'd found in one of our local supermarkets. The suitcases were definitely stylish, and the kids, especially Lucy, were impressed.

Clothing then. We were going from almost the end of a hot Greek summer to the end of a Christchurch winter. Knowing my city's reputation for its changeable four-seasons-in-one day climate, I had to be prepared for all types of weather. Hot here, balmy Singapore, the possibility of snow in New Zealand. Pat solved the problem of carrying cumbersome winter jackets as she borrowed a selection for the kids. Yanni's clothes were straightforward. He'd shopped in the UK and really needed only trainers. Lucy had amassed quite a wardrobe over the past few months and had a good choice, I wasn't too worried about my clothes but the twins ... ah, the twins. I had to buy clothes and shoes for Tony and Sam, who couldn't possibly travel in the hip-hop things they were wearing. Airport officials would baulk, wouldn't let us in to the country, when they saw the oversized trousers hanging off their bottoms! Typically, the twins had disappeared to Athens for a few days to stay with their cousins, due to return to Rhodes two days before our departure.

I was beginning to feel panicky.

'Just calm down for goodness sake,' Sheila told me on the telephone. 'Stop worrying about the twins and their shoes. You'll have time when they get back.'

The boys arrived back Thursday evening and Friday morning Sheila called to invite all the kids to Lindos later in the day. I was reluctant, knowing too well my children's reaction to that idea.

I was wrong. Surprisingly, they all agreed to come with me. After work we jumped into my little Fiat and headed off to find Sheila and Natalie in her Sunburnt Arms bar.

'Hi my love,' said Natalie, 'want a whisky?' 'Oh no, I'm driving, I'll have a juice,' I replied. 'Oh, go on, have a small Scotch. You might need it!' she said.

I wondered what for, but the boys were already ordering Red Bulls and Lucy, perched on a high barstool, was sipping a long fruit juice so, with a bit of a sigh, I accepted the whisky and Coke she placed before me. It tasted good. I took a long sip as Sheila and Natalie took some carry-on bags out from behind the bar.

'Here Lucy, that's yours. Yannis, Tony, Sam? Here you are. Oh,

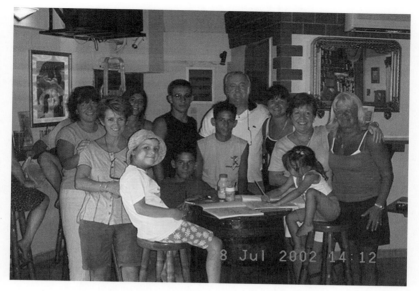

At the Sunburnt Arms in Lindos some weeks before our
journey to Christchurch: my friend Natalie is behind me,
her father Cliff is next to Yanni, and his wife
Rena is with Chris Sumner on the right

and here's yours Colleen,' Sheila said, putting a fifth brown pull-along
trolley bag beside me.

The children looked at the bags, at my friends, at me, at each other;
no one knew what to do. It was Natalie who broke the spell. 'Well, go
on then, open them!'

Lucy scrambled off the barstool and was quick to lie the bag flat,
unzipping and flipping the cover back. The boys did the same and all
four stepped back in surprise. Each travel bag was packed tight with
clothes, jackets, socks, shoes and a throwaway camera, everything,
including spending money.

I couldn't believe my eyes.

'Come on then, open yours, or maybe you should have another sip of
your drink first?' laughed Natalie.

'What on earth have you two done?'

'Nothing, we just wanted to help with your trip as well. You might
have to do some repacking though!'

My face wet with tears, I watched as Lucy and the boys tried on jackets, and coaxed me to rummage through what seemed to be an entire new wardrobe packed into a small suitcase. It was then I realised that we weren't alone in the bar. There were other people there and they were all smiling through teary eyes. The boys were laughing; Yannis checking out his new black Nikes, the twins comparing trousers and tops and trying new runners, which were a perfect fit. Lucy just sat back and smiled.

I couldn't do anything except hug my friends.

Sheila was smiling. 'I told you not to worry about their shoes didn't I? Thank goodness you listened to me for once!'

Monday 2 September

I'm sitting in the Departure lounge at Athens Airport watching as Yanni videos his sister watching the activity on the runway. Lucy's wearing a little crown, she's holding a magic wand and her wish is about to begin.

Early this morning, right on time, Gro pulled up outside the house in the Old Town in a shiny 4x4 truck. The kids laughed but we needed that vehicle to get us and all of our bags to the airport, where Sheila and Sharon were already waiting to see us off. It was like the start of an adventure, a wish; well, of course it was, it was Lucy's wish.

As always I was worried, about the Rebif (that, the very pleasant Aegean airline assistant assured me, would be taken care of by the staff after security clearance), about having forgotten something, about everything really. I needn't have been. Pam who was as compassionate, smiling and attractive as I had imagined from our telephone conversations met us in Athens. She produced the tickets, an envelope with Euros to cover our expenses and a special bag for Lucy – a pink pull-along packed with games and colouring books and crayons for the long journey.

'This is something extra for you Lucy. We think you're a princess so you deserve a special crown. And, of course, how can your wish come true without you having a magic wand!' Lucy's smile brought tears to Pam's eyes. 'You're a very special little girl who deserves something extraordinary. Now I wish I could join you just so I could see you and your Nana together.'

Standing up to leave, Pam smiled at me. 'I know this wish is going to go well. Have the best time and look after these wonderful children.' She left us in the capable hands of the Singapore Airlines' public relations officer, who ensured our check-in was trouble-free and my concerns over the injections unwarranted. My only worry was to remember to take the injections from the flight staff at the end of this leg of our journey.

3 or 4 September

(depending on where we are)

It's well after midnight and we are four or five hours into the flight from Singapore en route to my home town. Lucy is tucked up beside me sound asleep, her head on a pillow on the window seat armrest. Yannis is on my left and the twins are seated together across the aisle. It's quiet; there are just a few reading lights on. Even the twins have given up.

Our flight from Athens was an experience, to say the least. If I'd harboured any thoughts of doing what I had done on past long-haul flights – reading, watching films, and doing absolutely nothing for a change – I was an idiot. Once settled in our seats, either Lucy wanted to go to the toilet, couldn't work her sound system, wanted to swap places, wanted to go to sleep, wanted to watch the same movie as I was watching with her headsets, or the twins wanted one of the same things. Yanni was easy, settling quickly into the films and music; the twins, however, were on a high, determined to live this new experience of constant pampering from the attractive flight attendants. They ate all the airline food, clearing their trays and accepting every snack that was offered on what seemed an hourly basis. As all the passengers settled to snooze in the packed Boeing cabin the twins were bathed in light, heads down over a computer game, swaying together, listening to music. They didn't stop and when they weren't laughing over something, they were fighting over the game controls. More than once I had to hurry from my seat to separate them, which was unsettling and damned annoying, until Yanni got fed up and split them up.

We landed at Singapore before 6am, a beautiful Changi Airport representative waiting to direct us to a taxi shuttle to a downtown hotel. Lucy and the boys were a picture as we were directed through the mind-boggling airport. They didn't know where to turn, what to look at first, and when they weren't ogling the constant stream of mainly Asian passengers, they were jostling one another with surprise and delight.

Our taxi from the airport prompted a stunned silence that Tony broke five minutes into the journey. 'Wow, this is amazing Mum. But there's something I don't get. This taxi is older than any of the cabs on Rhodes, we should be rattling about, but it's like we're gliding along this road.'

'Idiot,' said his older brother. 'We're driving all right; the difference between here and Rhodes is that there are no potholes.' We all laughed. There were no potholes, just as there was no rubbish, no papers or empty cigarette packets clinging to the gutters. The roadside gardens and greenery were lush and immaculate.

We checked into a comfortable hotel minutes from the city centre, and were shown to a large room with two double beds and one single. There was a momentary scuffle over who would get the single bed; Yanni won of course. My insistence on a snooze after the long flight was met with a chorus of complaints, but within minutes I was the only one awake, lying next to Lucy and wondering what the journey had in store for us. I also slept for an hour or so, until the boys woke me, insistent on exploring Singapore. Yanni wanted to go to the zoo, Lucy wasn't keen, and I sensed an argument looming. I'd seen Singapore's Sentosa Island from a distance on previous trips and suggested an outing there. Yanni was not impressed but we went anyway, taking a taxi from the hotel to the HarbourFront MRT Station, which was under refurbishment. A cable car ride across the harbour gave us mind-boggling views of the city and its skyline.

We were on the resort island for more than three hours, posing in front of the famed Merlion statue, walking to some attractions and using the super-efficient monorail to access others. An observation tower on the site of a quirky historical museum provided a panoramic view of the city. Just when we'd all had about enough surprises and new experiences, we visited the island's underwater world, with its travelator moving us between every imaginable kind of fish, sea turtles and menacing sharks. There we posed for a fun photo before clambering into the cable car and riding past the harbour front to its higher Mount Faber station, which was also under reconstruction.

Reactions to Singapore? Yanni was conservative bordering on unenthusiastic (possibly tired but not prepared to admit it), the twins were ecstatic in their praise of everything and Lucy said she didn't like the smells.

'What smells?' 'All the smells!'

A deep breath. The day had been a far cry from my Singapore stopovers of lazing in the quiet hotel bed, window shopping on Orchard Road and soaking in a long hot bubble bath reading the Singapore *Straits Times*. My determination to retain that particular craving was shattered by Sam who, in typical twin-like fashion, had managed to clog the toilet. Try as I might I couldn't relax in that frothy tub; nor could I stop my children's hooting laughter.

The flight from Singapore to Christchurch was a milder version of the earlier leg. The kids knew what to expect and they were calmer … well, a bit. Tony and Sam continued to try whatever the cabin crew offered and seemed determined to finish every available game. At one stage their overhead lights were the only ones on in the Boeing cabin. Lucy was fine. She was small enough to curl up in her seat and slept like a kitten until the cloudy line of New Zealand's South Island was visible through the aircraft window. From then on she, Yanni and the twins were glued to the window, or they were at the larger viewing window near the toilets. I'd told the boys about flying over the Southern Alps into Christchurch's Airport, but they'd mocked my description.

'Yeah, sure Mum … we can just imagine all the snow-covered mountain peaks forming the backbone of your island, poking up through masses of clouds. Sounds like poetry, or you've been reading too many travel articles again!'

Now they nudged one another in silent awe at the magnificent landscape that was showing clearly below them.

Preparations for landing and the 'Fasten Seatbelts' sign pried the boys from the viewing window. The Boeing slowed and turned towards the terminal; my children were just about still sitting in their seats.

Welcome home Coll. Welcome to your other home, Lucy, Yanni, Tony and Sam.

Thursday 12 September

To put the past week or so into a few lines I must stretch whatever writing talents I have to the limit. Physical descriptions are relatively easy, and I can use Lucy and the boys' words to describe their surroundings: different, green, cars definitely on the 'wrong' side of the road, bungalow houses, gardens, wide streets, rivers, ducks and willow trees and fat woolly sheep.

Emotions are harder, touching the beginning and end of a scale that starts with Lucy's love for her grandmother and ends with her realisation that this is likely to be the only time they will spend together. This journey is not just Lucy's wish; it's also a dream.

Walking into the Arrivals hall after an effortless immigration check, the boys and Lucy's first impressions of Christchurch centred on a perky beagle that was busy sniffing bags and luggage for drugs and any foodstuffs that, by New Zealand law, had to be declared. The likeable little fellow didn't come near our mound of baggage and brown carry-ons, leaving the twins rather disappointed.

The welcome on the other side of the hall was overwhelming and emotional. Pat and her partner Trish knew the children from a visit to Rhodes a few years ago. For my nephew Nathan it was his first meeting with his Greek cousins. They were family and it showed; within minutes the boys, Nathan included, were teasing one another and Lucy was outnumbered as usual, and loving it.

Walking to the cars Pat took her niece's hand. 'Okay Lucy, you're the boss. This is your wish and you have to tell us what you want to do. We can go home now and you guys can relax a bit or we can go straight to see Nana.'

'I want to go to Nana.'

So we did, the two cars pulling into the grounds of Nazareth House 15 minutes later. Pat and Nathan parked opposite a bay window that looked out on to well-kept grass and garden.

I couldn't see if Mum was looking out waiting for us, but I imagined she was and wondered what her thoughts would be – what other elderly residents of this residential care home would think – watching the boys noisily scrambling out of Nathan's jeep and, in a subdued silence, leading Lucy into the main entrance.

Yanni insisted on catching Lucy's wish on video. I suspected he wanted to seem busy, and it was his way of coping with the emotions attached to the moment. His video expertise during our stay in Christchurch started and ended with my mother's, 'Hello, dear!'

That moment, when Lucy moved across Mum's small room to hug her frail grandmother, was something incredibly special, almost sacred. It was a bonding of grandmother and granddaughter who had never really known one another, whose conversations never went beyond a few words on the telephone. That moment erased the miles and years that had separated them.

It was magic. As Lucy gestured for her brothers to join her on and around her grandmother, it was exactly what Make A Wish had offered Lucy. It was her wish.

We settled into our temporary home next to Pat and Trish. The house was compact and contained a living room leading onto a small kitchen, doors off a hall leading to a bathroom and two bedrooms. Lucy and I were to share one room, the twins the other. Yanni had his own room on the garage level of Pat and Trish's split-level home. His discomfort and disappointment was obvious but Pat's reaction swift.

'Come on then. We've got a lilo in the storeroom. We can blow that up and you can stay with the twins.'

Yanni looked at his aunt. 'Blow up a lilo ...'

'Yeah a lilo! Well it's not really a lilo, it's an air mattress, a posh lilo if you like, Yanni. And we'll just blow it up and you can sleep on that.'

I translated into slow English and then Greek and Yanni relaxed. It was just one of the language traps my children floundered into. Thankfully they didn't last long and invariably ended in howls of laughter.

Pat's neighbours had thoughtfully stocked our little residence with basic necessities – bread, butter and biscuits in the kitchen, shampoo, soap and washing powder in the bathroom. We were all touched by their hospitality. The little house quickly became a cozy base for our daily visits with Mum and adventures that would undoubtedly remain etched in our minds forever.

Pat lent us her and Trish's car, a Toyota saloon. Roomy and luxurious, it seemed massive compared to my little Fiat Panda; it was also automatic. That, combined with the thought of driving on the left-hand side of the road again after so long, had me worrying about my ability to take the kids out. I dreaded negotiating the rather tight twist in and out of the parking space. I didn't voice my uncertainties to the kids as any scoffing would have made me worse. The first time I took a deep breath, got in, started up and took off, realising that without the car we would be dependent on Pat, who was working much of the time, or public transport.

Thanks Pat. Your car was great.

Every morning and evening we would descend en masse on Nazareth House. Mum would be waiting for us, as would many of her housemates, the nuns and the nursing staff, who obviously enjoyed the liveliness of the kids in that normally subdued atmosphere.

'Morning, kalimera!' the boys would call at whoever had buzzed them through from the reception desk. Flashing big smiles, they would rush in for hugs with their grandmother before heading further down the passageway to the residents' playroom, which they'd discovered on the first day. They liked the idea that their quietly spoken Nana sometimes played at the pool table. She had told them that 'your grandfather and I were pretty hot pool players in our time,' and she'd laughed at the boys' quizzical reaction. 'We weren't always this old you know!' Of course, they coaxed Mum into showing them her skills. 'Sam, check out the way Nana holds the cue,' said Tony, 'I'm impressed!'

Lucy was quieter; she preferred to sit with her Nana, who moved in her armchair to make way for her granddaughter. They were like two interlocking pieces of a jigsaw puzzle; a perfect fit.

Pat and Trish's comfortable home, hidden on a back section up a long driveway off a riverside avenue, was a quiet haven of good taste. Both

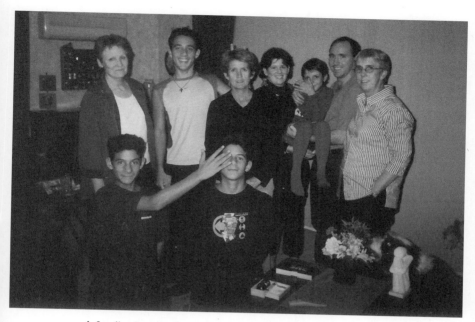

A family shot: back row from left Trish (Pat's partner), Yanni, Colleen, Mel (my nephew's wife), Lucy, Nathan (my nephew) and my sister Pat; front row from left Sam and Tony

had older children who lived elsewhere, and the two professional women enjoyed the company of a dog named Polly and a cat named Bella. All four were used to a pretty quiet existence until we moved in next door.

The houses were separated by a small garage, with just a few short steps between the two front doors that my kids, especially the boys, rarely closed. They got into the habit of ringing Pat's doorbell every time they went in the front door. It scared the hell of out poor Bella, who from the second day of our residence took one look at the foursome from Rhodes and promptly hid herself in the laundry cupboard. Polly was a wonderful cross between a Springer spaniel and a bearded collie but she didn't act like a dog; she was part of the family and part of the Rhodian quartet whenever they ding-danged their way into Pat's comfy and relaxed home.

Some evenings we went out. My school friend Marg threw a barbecue, inviting mutual friends and their children to meet my new and old family at her eye-catching wooden home, precariously perched on high stilts on the hillside. We feasted on New Zealand mussels, sausages and salads, and drank good local wine, while the kids made the most of the full-size trampoline in Marg's yard. They took turns, laughing and jumping until one friend's unstoppable little son bounced too high, too wide and disappeared over the dividing fence. That calmed them all down a bit.

Most evenings were spent at Pat and Trish's, or walking Polly along the willow-tree lined riverbank to the local park and later feeding the ducks from the bridge across the muddy Heathcote River. Meals varied from a mouth-watering parcel wrapped in paper, a $12 feast from the local fish and chip shop, to Chinese takeaways, Kentucky Fried Chicken, and other healthier food produced by my sister and her ever patient, ever smiling partner. Trish was a music teacher and she sat with Lucy at the piano and taught her to play *Happy Birthday* while the boys listened to more interruptive music.

Some evenings I worried about Yanni, who was increasingly remote and spent too long in the toilet next door. He was getting thinner and I suspected was bordering on bulimic. Pat noticed as well, but my enquiries made him moody so I decided to broach the subject on our return to Rhodes.

We'd been fortunate. Spending 24 hours a day together for the first time in many years could have been a disaster. However, the bad moments were few compared to the highlights of the journey.

Besides driving the kids up and around the Port Hills to give them a panoramic view of my home town and its amazing setting between the Pacific Coast and the flat Canterbury Plains that end dramatically in mountain ranges, one of our first adventures was ice-skating. All four children had tried rollerblades but ice was totally new and, to be honest, I started to regret my decision as soon as Lucy was impatiently demanding that her skates be tied. What if she fell? What if someone knocked her over? What if she got hurt? I was too worried about the 'what ifs' to see her glide away on Yanni's arm. She wobbled a bit but didn't fall, and looked a natural within minutes.

We drove out of the city with Nathan and his wife Mel, towards the mountains, to spend hours on a sheep and ostrich farm where Lucy and Yanni bottle-fed the chubby lambs and the twins dug their fingers deep into the thick coats of merino sheep. The friendly farmer whisked

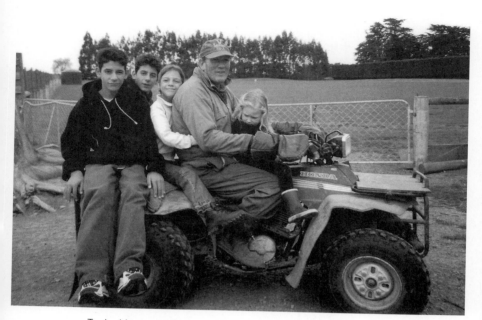

Tucked between Sam and Tony and the West Melton farmer,
Lucy looked totally at ease, a picture of health and happiness

the kids around his property on a hefty four-wheeler; Lucy's face was a picture of health and freedom. Nathan joined us go-carting and Lucy cried because she was not allowed to join her brothers. Her tantrum was cut short by our near hysterical laughter at the boys' antics on the track.

Ten-pin bowling with Marg and her two teenage boys proved a great success and we agreed to go to Christchurch's Queen Elizabeth II swimming complex the next day, where Yanni and Lucy bodysurfed fake waves and the skinny, spindly-legged twins left muscly tough-looking Maori kids shaking their heads in disbelief as they dived off the highest diving board.

The next day we'd planned to drive north of Christchurch to Hanmer Springs, a popular alpine spa area known for its hot sulphur pools and a range of more lively attractions. Determined to match the twins' daring diving, Yanni said he would bungee jump off a bridge en route to Hanmer. I knew the jump site well and had vivid memories of the historic bridge that spanned the muddy waters of the Waiau River; it had been a spot Dad always stopped at on frequent family trips to

Hanmer as it offered magnificent views towards the rugged mountains surrounding the Waiau Gorge. I was sure Yanni would not jump.

'You won't do it,' I insisted.

'Wannabet'?

I laughed at how quickly Yanni had picked up the New Zealand habit of running words together. 'Yeah, I'll bet you.'

'How much?

'How much do you have?'

'I still have the 50 Euros from your friends in Lindos. So that's 100 New Zealand dollars!' The twins and Lucy were nudging one another.

'Okay, you're on.'

It had the makings of quite a day. I had hired an eight-seater minivan so Pat and Trish could join us in one vehicle and Marg, her sister and their families arranged to meet us in Hanmer. We arrived at Yanni's proposed jump site after a 90-minute drive and, looking at the bridge and the 35-metre drop, I was sure he would change his mind.

I was wrong. While Pat, Trish and the twins waited for Yanni at the lookout spot, coffee shop and tourist centre just before the bridge, Lucy insisted that she and I accompany her brother on to the bridge. The bungee operators worked from the centre of the bridge, where a friendly young man introduced himself and explained to Yanni what he should and shouldn't do. Lucy was laughing at first, but as Steve fastened the bungee rope around Yanni's ankles and he moved out on to a small platform she grabbed my hand and squeezed, hard.

Listening carefully to Steve's instructions, Yanni's face was a strange combination of daring and dread.

'Just reach out opposite, Yanniise, like you're going to touch those trees over there.'

Yanni turned and looked at us with a 'What the hell?' expression, turned back to face the trees on the left bank opposite the bridge and, on the order of 'One, two, three bungee!' dived off the platform.

Lucy and I gasped and then laughed as a cry of 'Mum, my shoes!' echoed around us. We watched as Yanni sprang back towards the bridge, only to hurtle down once again to the quick moving waters of the river below. As his movement slowed, a speedboat moved to catch Yanni and take him to the riverbank where he ran up to meet us at the observation point.

He was beaming, and quick to remind me that I had lost the bet, owed him $100 and yes, he would take up his aunty's offer to purchase an 'I Bungeed' t-shirt. Lucy and the twins were impressed and Yanni held court on the 15-minute drive into Hanmer town centre. Waiting for Marg and her sister we played minigolf, then we crossed the road to the thermal pools and spa, which proved a far cry from the rather off-putting pools of my childhood memories. There were more than 10 pools to choose from and I believe we tried them all. Lucy was not keen on the hotter pools, which didn't seem to suit me either.

'I'd get out of there if I was you,' Pat advised as I lounged in one of the hot rocky tubs. 'You look a bit like a lobster!' The complex included waterslides that Lucy and Marg's niece had to be dragged away from as we headed to the Hanmer domain for a picnic lunch. There the boys tried their hand at cricket while the adults sat and relaxed. Heading out of town we stopped at a maze, which had everyone in fits of laughter, and then it was into the cars and on the road home. The only stop was at a famed ice cream shop where, sitting in a line along the gutter, we all got into terrible messes eating delicious chocolate-dipped ice creams.

It was a full and memorable day, as was the next when we took a train across the South Island to the West Coast, passing through long tunnels and seeing dramatic mountain scenery. Unusually there was little snow en route and sadly a bitterly cold and consistent drizzle dashed any plans of exploring the former centre of New Zealand's gold-rush days at the end of the tracks. We ate in a time-warped Greymouth diner and the train turned back towards Christchurch.

Another day I took the kids to a huge zoo, where we saw the nocturnal kiwi, giraffes, zebras, lions and ever-mischievous monkeys. Lucy ran wilder than the animals and, against my better judgment, insisted on trying the flying-fox tree swing. From there we went on to find my brother, Jim, at his house on the outskirts of the city. The kids loved the mad assortment of garden gnomes, knick-knacks and treasures that he and his wife, Wendy, had collected over the years. Lucy and the boys lolled on their king-size waterbed and later scoffed at my singing as Jim amazed them with a vast collection of karaoke equipment he used semi-professionally.

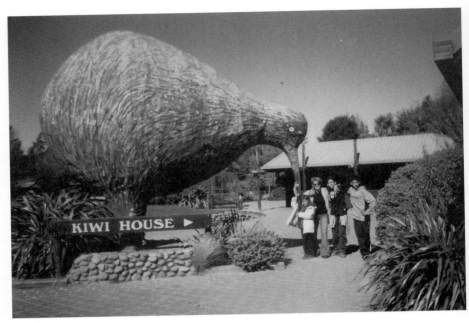

My "Greek Kiwis" were amazed to find real kiwis at Orana
Wildlife Park, with Yanni taking this shot of us near an
enlarged version of New Zealand's unique flightless bird
outside the Kiwi House

One freezing evening the boys went to a local rugby match with
Nathan and Mel, returning bright-cheeked from the rugby banter,
twirling noisy wooden rattles and mimicking the local crowd with their
Canterbury chanting.

Through all of this I injected Lucy with her Rebif every second day and
kept an eye on her neck. Only once did she look pale and off colour,
but whatever was bothering her was cured by a trip into the city to take
the Christchurch tram to the city's museum. We later hit the shops for
souvenirs, getting presents for Lucy's friends in Athens and on Rhodes.
We even found a small ceramic lamb for her doctor.

The injections, most days, were nightmares, taking much longer than
necessary. Lucy and I wandered around the small kitchen one day for an
hour like circling wrestlers, before she would let me jab her arm. 'Come

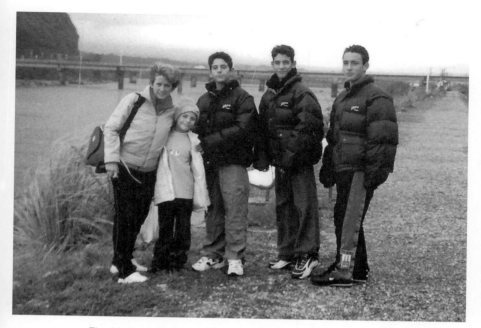

The Mortzos family at Greymouth: the jackets my friends in Lindos had surprised us with were needed on that bitterly cold but enjoyable outing on the TranzAlpine Express train from Christchurch to the West Coast

on Lucy; let's get it over and done with.' 'No I can't yet.' She started to cry. 'You don't know what it's like. It hurts, it stings; I can't do it yet.' Lucy had no idea how much it hurt me to do something that hurt her. But it had to be done and, in the end, she relented and the whole performance was promptly forgotten.

Leaving Christchurch was difficult. I won't describe the feelings as I know I will start to cry again. We left behind a Nana who, for my children, was no longer just a voice at the end of the telephone. We left family and friends and a city that had become a temporary home for my children.

Lucy's wish has been completed and I'm now wondering how we are going to settle back to normal everyday life on Rhodes.

It won't be easy for anyone.

Monday 16 September

I'm sitting next to Lucy on an Aegean Airlines flight from Athens to Rhodes. We arrived back in Athens very early this morning, after a long day and a half of travelling and flying. That return flight is always a killer. It's too long and all your body wants to do is fall into a large comfortable bed, not try to sleep upright in a slightly tilted airline seat.

We arrived dazed at Athens Airport, all knowing that a television crew would probably be waiting for us. (When we were organising the trip Make A Wish asked for permission to talk to Lucy at some stage. There were three choices: no contact whatsoever, limited contact, and full contact. I chose limited and had agreed that a television channel could approach us at some stage.) I didn't really expect them to be waiting as we left the Arrivals hall, bleary-eyed and extremely tired. They had arranged for us to go for breakfast at the airport hotel, which was better than waiting in the airport, but still all we wanted to do was relax and sleep. Lucy wouldn't look at them. She flew at me, hit out, hit me and bit me.

Oh dear.

Welcome back to Greece.

I wanted to talk to them, tell them all about Make A Wish, but Lucy wouldn't let me do anything. The television crew left, dejected and without their spot, and we flew on to Rhodes.

Back to life, back to reality.

Wednesday 18 September

Back to work for me, back to school for Lucy, a new technical senior high school for the twins and, sadly, disappointment for Yanni, who wasn't accepted into the chef school to which he had applied.

Yanni is a mess. He's thin and hardly eating anything. When he does eat I am sure he is making himself sick soon afterwards. I tried to talk with him but he is unapproachable, saying only that he knows what he is doing, that he is in control of his body, but I wonder. As soon as Lucy and I return from Athens I think I will try to get professional help, before he turns anorexic. On one subject he is strong and adamant. He says he will resit his national exams and go to Athens University sports academy. He does not want to settle for less.

This morning I called TAO and arranged for blood tests for Lucy on the 24th. That should also be the final Rebif prescription and the end, I hope, of any medication for Lucy.

The end of her struggle with cancer, and the beginning of coping after cancer ...

Wednesday 25 September

Athens was effortless as far as Lucy's blood tests and her final prescription were concerned. She was full of stories of her Nana and of her journey, confident and laughing with her doctor. As she presented him with the ceramic lamb, she told him, 'While I was there I learned that New Zealand has millions and millions, something ridiculous, like 50 million sheep. Well, I got to know a couple of the little ones and they looked just like this.' She was quite a different girl. The tests were fine and I was able to get the final injections without any hassles, running to and from the Athens city centre without having time to think about how it was all coming to an end.

Little Dimitri was in the clinic, in a room on his own again. Smaro had brightened it up with some of his favourite things, among them a Harry Potter poster and postcards from Lucy. Smaro was, as always, at his bedside, welcoming us with open arms and a brave smile. Dimitri couldn't talk, he just grinned when he saw Lucy as she moved Smaro's chair close to her sick little friend. Dimitri turned his head slightly so he could see Lucy and their eyes locked. For a moment I thought Lucy was overwhelmed by the situation and I questioned my own insistence on seeing Dimitri. But I was wrong, she was simply Lucy, an eight year-old who loved her friend and wanted him to share her wish.

She wove a story about her Nana and her cousins, feeding lambs, bubbling in a hot pool, eating chocolate-dipped ice creams, running through the zoo and seeing a live kiwi. 'Funny little thing but really cute – just like you Dimitri!' His eyes sparkled and told her what he couldn't say.

'I found one just for you. Look, I'll put it here so you can see it and think of all those times we played together at Elpida.' Lucy placed the small souvenir on his bedside cabinet, reached over and lightly hugged her friend.

'We have to go now and I'll see you when I come for my next tests. Okay Dimitri, you'll be here waiting for me, right?'

Smaro was smiling, but her eyes were glazed; she was sad and scared and there was nothing I could say or do to help her.

I can't believe that this little boy will die. Not Dimitri.

Leaving TAO to head to the airport we bumped into Alexandros, who was waiting for his mother to finish with medical insurance payments in another part of the hospital. He was as bouncy and as cheeky as ever, full of life and complaints that Lucy couldn't spend more time with him.

'Next time!' Lucy shouted as we ran down the 'smoking terrace' steps and left Alexandros grinning and waving at the main door.

I am back on Rhodes with mixed feelings. Lucy's test results were outstanding and we don't have to go back until March, but what about all those children we left behind? Lucy's getting back into her life, full of life and confidence; she's picking up where she left off ...

But what of our little friends' lives? What of their parents?

What future will they have?

Thursday 17 October

I was at work when Stella called.

Brave perky Stella, pregnant with another baby after all she had been through with little Panayiotis.

'I thought you would want to know, knowing how close you are to Smaro,' she said.

I didn't want to hear what she had to say. I wanted to close the phone.

'Dimitri died today. Colleen, are you there? Did you hear me?'

Dimitri wasn't the last of our friends to die. We lost Magda, Antony, Alexandros, Vaso, and other children from the hostel, from the clinic.

They have all gone.

Lucy is here.